Getting Back to <u>BASICS</u>

"What your doctor wanted to tell you... <u>but didn't have the time"</u>

<u>Second Edition</u>

Barry M. Stein, D.P.E.
Clinical Exercise Physiologist

Get Fit For Life, LLC
Bayside, New York 11360
(718) 541-4508
www.MyTrueAge.com

Comments/Suggestions
bmstein@gmail.com

Getting Back to BASICS

"What your doctor wanted to tell you...
but didn't have the time"

Second Edition

First Edition   - Copyright 2001 Barry M. Stein
Second Edition - Copyright 2009 Barry M. Stein

All right reserved. Printed in the United States of America. No part of this publication may be reproduced, stored in a retrieval system or transmitted in any form or by any means, electronically, mechanically, photocopying, recording or otherwise, without the written permission of the publisher.

Printed in the United States of America

ISBN 978-0-615-27739-4

Publisher:
Get Fit For Life, LLC
2642 202 Street
Bayside, New York 11360-2325
bmstein@gmail.com

Table of Contents

Part 1 -	**A Wake-Up Call**	1
	• *Some Unexpected News*	3
Part 2 -	**Control Your Risk Factors**	9
	• *The BASICS For Staying Healthy*	11
	• *How Old Are You Really?*	14
Part 3 -	**The Weight Management Dilemma**	17
	• *The Obesity Epidemic*	19
	• *Eat Right To Stay Healthy*	23
	• *Some Food For Thought*	31
Part 4 -	**Exercise: Essential, Not Optional**	37
	• *Exercise Promotes Better Health*	39
	• *Develop A Healthy Heart*	44
	• *Sensible Guidelines For Resistance Training*	51
	• *Keep Well Hydrated: Drink Water*	56
	• *Stretching May Prevent Injuries*	58
Part 5 -	**Manage Stress To Stay Healthy**	59
	• *The Mind/Body Connection*	61
	• *Manage Stress Or Suffer Distress*	64
	• *Keep Your Sense Of Humor*	70
Part 6 -	**The Importance Of A Good Nights Sleep**	75
	• *Sleep Soundly*	77
	• *10-Tips For Better Sleep*	79
	• *Sleep Problems In Children*	80
Part 7 -	**The Unlikely Piece Of The Wellness Puzzle**	81
	• *Manage Your Money To Stay Healthy*	83
	• *The Impact Of Today's Economy On Your Health*	89
Part 8 -	**Putting The Pieces Together**	91
	• *There Are No Excuses*	93
	• *So Now You Know*	100
Appendix A	**Resistance-Training Program**	103
Appendix B	**About The Author**	120

Introduction

Getting Back to BASICS is intended as a guide for healthful living. My goal in writing this book was to bring together, under one umbrella, some useful information, which may help you to more thoroughly enjoy your life. The information presented in this book is intended to support the recommendations of your personal physician. It should not be considered a substitute for their sound medical advice.

When the First Edition of ***Getting Back to BASICS*** was completed in 2001 life was very different. Over the past eight years we've witnessed a budget surplus become a crushing deficit and an escalation in world tension materially change our lives. We've also seen a significant increase in health problems, including an unparalleled rise in adult and childhood obesity. It appears we're moving in the wrong direction. Now, more than ever, *'we must focus our attention on making healthy choices to meet the stressful demands of our increasing complex world.'*

> To my wonderful wife, Lenore and loving daughters, Deborah and Shana. Their inspiration, support and encouragement made this book a reality. And to Ashley, the best little reader in our family.

Book Cover: Dice Garcia, Venture Promotions
Website Design: Jason C. Weber

Editing
Lenore Stein
Shana Stein

Professional Review

Nancy Copperman, MS, RD, CDN
Director of Public Health Initiatives
North Shore-Long Island Jewish Health System

Christine Megan, PhD
Clinical Psychologist
Center for Weight Management
North Shore-Long Island Jewish Health System

*'I'm not telling you it's going to be easy ...
I'm telling you it's going to be worth it'*
Art Williams

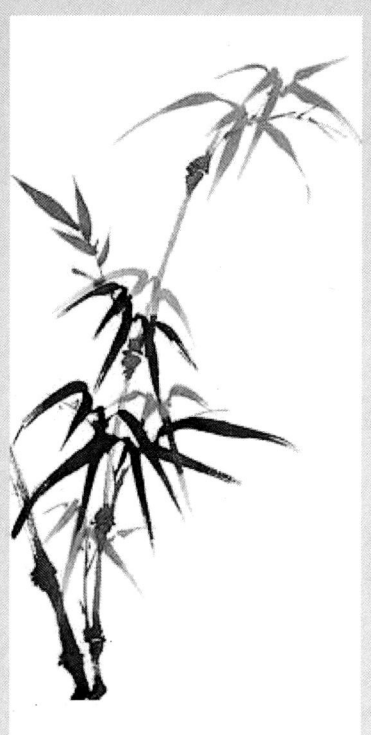

Part 1

A Wake-Up Call

Some Unexpected News

The New Reality

The start of the current recession in December 2007 marked the beginning of a new reality for the majority of Americans. As the economic bubble burst we began to realize that life, as we knew it, was about to change. Up until that date, most Americans believed everything was possible, and that we could live _the good life_, giving little thought to possible consequences.

Today, we live the new reality. Consumers have been forced to cut back on spending. They've stopped buying cars, purchasing homes and have been forced to postpone vacations - as they see their retirement savings decline, home values plummet and unemployment rise. It almost appears as if we awoke from a pleasant dream to a less than pleasant almost _nightmarish_ reality.

Let's take a moment to compare life before the recession and life today

	January 2007 (Pre-Recession)	March 2009 (Recession)
Dow Jones Industrial Average	12,114.10	7,170.06
Unemployment rate	4.6 %	10.1 %
Number of Unemployed	7 million	11.6 million
People on Food Stamps	26.3 million	31.1 million
Annual Personal Bankruptcy Filings	823,405	1,504,634
Monthly Home Foreclosures	148,425	274,399
Number of Homes Sold	7.3 million	4.8 million
Median Home Price	$211,000	$170,300
Value of Americans' 401(k) Savings	$2.7 trillion	$2.4 trillion
Credit Card Debt	$902.3 billion	$994.4 billion

Data Sources: Department of Labor, Department of Agriculture, Mortgage Bankers Association, National Association of Realtors, FDIC, Federal Reserve, Employee Benefit Research Institute, Treasury Department

How Do We Cope With This New Reality? We recognize that the economic conditions today, bring new stressors, which require us to reinforce the foundation upon which we structure our lives. We reflect back to a simpler time, focusing on products and ideas, which have time-tested reliability, as we direct our attention towards ...

Getting Back to BASICS.

Some Unexpected News

You've just completed your annual physical exam and you're sitting in your doctor's office waiting to hear the results. You're a little apprehensive because you've noticed that you haven't been feeling as good as you usually do. You're not sleeping well and your weight has been steadily rising. You're thinking back to the time when your father said, *'as you get older you have to expect those little aches and pains.'* That was three years before his heart attack. As you sit there, you begin to worry that your fate is sealed, that there's nothing you can do to prevent the inevitable.

In walks Dr. Walker. His expression, difficult to read, sends a chill up your spine. That ache in the pit of your stomach tells you that things are not what they should be. The only question that remains is - <u>*how bad are they?*</u> Suddenly that comfortable chair you've been sitting in becomes rock hard. Your body shifts side-to-side, your back straightens as your muscles tighten. You lean forward as you strain to listen to what he has to say.

'Your test results came back normal.'

Immediately the floodgates of emotion burst open as you feel a wave of renewed energy fill your body and soul. Comfortably you settle back into your chair to hear the remainder of his report. Yet, somewhere deep in the recesses of your mind you can't help but feel that once again, *'you've dodged the bullet.'*

As you continue to listen, you find yourself doing what you usually do when the doctor says everything is *'okay.'* The emotion of the moment has you so exhilarated, that your mind wanders and you don't pay close attention to what he's saying.

'Bob, you better listen carefully to this,' he says.

The words jolt your body back to consciousness as if you were abruptly awakened from a pleasant dream.

'What's the problem?' you ask. *'I thought you said the results were normal.'*

'They are, but things can change - and usually do - if you don't begin to get back to basics.'

'What do you mean get back to basics, Dr. Walker?'

'It means learning to make changes in your life that may help you to keep those test results normal.'

'Just tell me what to do and I'll do it,' you say.

'It's not that simple, Bob. It means developing a different lifestyle than the one you're accustomed to.'

'Well, just tell me what to do and I'll do it,' you repeat.

'Unfortunately, it's not that easy. Most doctors, myself included, don't have the time to chat about getting back to basics. We're so busy treating patients and handling our practice that we just don't have the time to properly counsel patients on how to make positive lifestyle changes. While I can tell you what you should and shouldn't be doing, I don't have time to go into lengthy explanations.'

'If you can't give me guidance, then how am I supposed to learn what to do?'

'I have a book I'd like you to read. Many of the things I would say to you, if I had the time, are explained in this book.'

'If you think it will help, I'll read it.'

'Yes I do, Bob. In fact, I think you should read it several times.'

"It's that important?"

'Let's put it this way, Bob. Almost every day we hear about miracle drugs, nutritional supplements and new advances in the field of Anti-Aging Medicine. People have come to expect that they can pop a pill to stay healthy. Honestly speaking, how can someone who smokes, drinks and overeats expect to find the fountain of youth in a pill or an injection? My suggestion to you is to read the book and if you still have questions, I'll be happy to discuss them with you.'

On the way home that day, you feel a sense of peace that the test results came back normal. You remember rushing to tell your wife Audrey the good news only to find her sitting quietly in the living room.

'What's wrong?' you say, sensing that something was terribly amiss.

'The office called,' she said.

'What's wrong?' you repeat.

'They said that Bill had a heart attack at work today.'

'How is he?'

'He didn't make it to the hospital in time.'

You feel the blood drain from your face as your throat tightens. You and Bill had lunch yesterday afternoon in the diner across the street from work. He looked to be in perfect health, no sign of any problem. You remember him saying to you that he intended to stop smoking as you discussed your future retirement plans. After all, you're both baby boomers and nearing retirement age. *How could it be? How could he be gone? ... Why?*

Your knees buckle as you sit down. Your wife comes over to hug you and you both sit quietly for many minutes.

'How did your checkup go?' she finally asked.

'Oh, the results were normal. I'm fine.'

'I'm so happy,' she said.

As you sat there contemplating the untimely death of your colleague and friend, you begin to think about your own mortality. You and Bill had a lot in common - you ate poorly, smoked, hated to exercise and were overweight. At that moment you realized that if you didn't change, you might be next. Dr. Walker was right. You needed to make some serious lifestyle changes right now. If you wanted to continue to stay healthy, you had to learn how to get back to basics.

This story begins on the sidewalks of any town or city in America just at the end of World War II. The climate of the country was changing from the fears, frustrations and uncertainties of a wartime economy, to one based on guarded optimism for the future. No longer were there any doubts in the minds of most Americans that the world they knew was changing, hopefully for the better. This renewed sense of optimism for a bright future, helped fuel the sudden and dramatic increase in childbirths which has come to be known as the baby boomer generation.

It was a cold, windy day in New York when a fragile child was born to a young couple at the Madison Park Hospital in Brooklyn. The date was September 30, 1947. At first everything appeared to be normal, as a healthy baby boy, the newest edition to the baby boomer generation was delivered. Soon after the birth it became apparent that everything was not all right, something was terribly wrong. This tiny infant, unable to feed properly, was choking with every attempt. The diagnosis confirmed the worst fears of those involved. This innocent victim of life, barely one day old, was born with a serious birth defect. His trachea (*windpipe*) and esophagus (*food tube*) were joined. As this tiny newborn attempted to swallow milk, this life giving sustenance was filling his lungs. The very liquid meant to nourish this new life was drowning it.

Time was running out. The only way this baby could survive would be to undergo an extensive operation to separate his trachea and esophagus. To make matters worse, the only hospital that had experience with this new surgical procedure was in Boston, Massachusetts. In spite of the odds, some means were found to have that innocent, helpless victim flown to Boston for surgery the following day at Boston Children's Hospital.

October 1st, 1947 was a tough day for the new arrival as he underwent a lengthy and dangerous operation. Thankfully, that fragile bundle of flesh, completely oblivious to the turmoil surrounding him, survived the surgery and showed the world something that day. He wasn't giving up on life, and that in spite of the staggering odds against him, he had strength, determination - *he was a survivor*.

As the years passed, that fragile newborn grew into a healthy young man, never fully understanding why some people, often people he did not know, would refer to him as the '*miracle baby*.' It took quite some time for that baby boomer to realize how fortunate he truly was.

It boggles the mind to think that in the span of just two days, so many correct decisions had to be made. Dr. Sidney Thier, the family's doctor and personal friend, had to make the correct diagnosis and arrange transportation to Boston Children's Hospital in a timely manner. And, Dr. Paul Lowenstein had to use remarkable skill in performing this radically new surgical procedure. Perhaps most of all, that tiny fragile newborn, the newest member of the baby boomer generation, had to muster all of his strength, determination and '*will-to-live*' in order to beat the odds against him.

All of those things, and so many other pieces of the puzzle, had to blend in perfect harmony in order to bring about a successful conclusion. Yet, in spite of the odds against that happening, no delays took place, no errors were made and the '*miracle baby*' survived and prospered. Only now, after so many years have passed, can one fully understand and appreciate the significance of those first few days of - **MY LIFE**.

That's right, I was (*am*) that fragile '*miracle baby*.' While I have no direct memories of that episode in my life, I bear the extensive scars that remain, as a badge of courage. Over the years, I have come to realize that my life, to this point, has been an experiment, to see what works for me - and what doesn't. Through my studies, personal life and clinical experience, I have come to realize that good health, doesn't just happen. In order to stay healthy, you must make a personal commitment to get back to basics and make healthy lifestyle choices.

Most people consciously or unconsciously wrote me off that fateful day, October 1st 1947. Still others probably never expected me to return to New York six months later. I am certain that many others, who knew me from birth, never expected me to grow up, become happily married and the proud father of two beautiful daughters. Whenever someone referred to me as the '*miracle baby*' while I was growing up, they were probably thinking, '*I never expected that kid to survive.*' Happily, I proved them wrong and as a bona fide member of the baby boomer generation, I intend to continue to prove them wrong for a very long time.

Having given you some insight into the nature of the author, I can say that, in spite of my health problems, or possibly because of them, I have gained a greater appreciation for life, family, friends and good health. I believe that because I have struggled for so long to become healthy, I can say with complete certainty that the old adage is true, *'that one only comes to appreciate their health when he or she loses it.'* But, having lost it, and thereafter regained it - that is a special gift, a second chance to appreciate the most valuable personal asset you will ever have your good health.

While I have been involved in the field of Wellness for more than thirty years, I must admit right up front that the majority of information I write about in this book was not invented or thought up by me. Most of the advice I offer was written about, or presented by others - in some cases long before I or any member of the baby boomer generation was born. So why write the book? Simply, to bring together under one umbrella some valuable ideas that may help you to more fully enjoy your life.

This brings me to a second critically important point. As you read this book, you must understand that *the advice I offer may not be valid for everyone*. While we have a great many similarities anatomically and physiologically, we all have subtle differences that make us who we are. I recognize that the age and current health status of each reader may vary widely. A particular exercise suggestion or food recommendation may be appropriate for one person and not be advisable for another. With this in mind,

I caution all readers to consult with their doctor and have a complete medical examination prior to implementing any suggestion or recommendation made in this book.

As I bring this opening chapter to a close, I would like to relate an interesting story, which makes an appropriate point.

It seems that, almost every morning on my way to work I would drive down a certain street and see a man standing outside of his home either washing or waxing his car. The car wasn't a new car. In fact, it looked to be at least nine or ten years old. As I drove past this man I often marveled at his dedication to keeping his car in such fine condition. Standing outdoors in all types of weather, rag in hand, polishing and grooming this old, but not antique car.

One day I took a closer look at the man. His age appeared to be about fifty, maybe a little older. His head was balding and his stomach was protruding well over the belt buckle of his blue jeans. While he held a rag in one hand, his other hand usually held a lit cigarette. Obviously, this man was not a great physical specimen. I had seen many out-of-shape men just like him. Why then was the picture of this man exhibiting such compulsive behavior troubling me?

Finally, it came to me, and surprisingly, the answer came from the lessons I learned during my earliest days in grammar school. I had always been taught that the human body was like a machine. Treat it right and it would last a long time. Treat it poorly and it would break down. At that moment I realized what was bothering me. As I traveled down that particular street each morning, what I was actually seeing was a snapshot of how many of us treat our health. This vivid picture highlighted the fact that many of us, while neglecting our health, place undo importance on other tasks. This overweight, sedentary, pencil-pushing smoker symbolized in my mind how misplaced our priorities have become. Here was a man, compulsively washing and waxing an old car, who obviously needed to make some serious lifestyle changes, In a sense, he was the one who truly needed the fresh coat of paint with an engine overhaul. It struck me as tragically funny when I finally realized that, an alarming number of us, treat our <u>cars</u> better than we treat our <u>health</u>.

If you're reading this book, you've probably been told to do so by your doctor or on the recommendation of a friend or relative. For whatever reason, they believe that you need to consider making some basic lifestyle adjustments in order to stay healthy. While you might not agree with them, I hope that while you read this book <u>you keep an open mind.</u>

Just because your doctor said that you have to make some lifestyle adjustments, it's not the end of the world. You should think of it as a new beginning. If you're honest with yourself, you know that you haven't exactly been following a healthy lifestyle. Chances are you haven't been feeling good and this should serve as a wake up call for change. So what's the problem? You don't know how to change? No problem that's what this book is all about. Teaching you how to develop a healthy lifestyle by…

Getting Back to <u>BASICS</u>.

You probably should consider yourself very lucky. Most of the time people wait until it's too late. I'm sure you could tell me a story about an acquaintance that didn't make it to the hospital in time. That's because *'the effects of an unhealthy lifestyle are cumulative. Heart attacks and strokes are culminating events that follow years of personal neglect.'*

As I bring this first chapter to a close, I want to remind you of something you already know. The story I mentioned earlier highlights the unfortunate fact that many of us place undo importance on '*things*' at the expense of our health. We all know, maintaining good health is much more important than any physical possession. It sounds so simple, '*yet each day millions of us place our health at great risk as we strive for greater wealth and possessions.*'

'Things change for the better when we take responsibility...
For our thoughts, decisions and actions'
Unknown

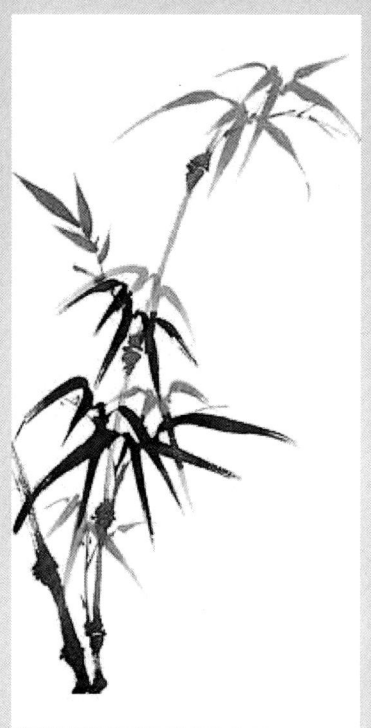

Part 2

Control Your Risk Factors

The BASICS For Staying Healthy

How Old Are You Really?

Risk Factors for Cardiovascular Disease

We all have risk factors, conditions or behaviors that increase our chance of getting certain diseases. Some risk factors for heart disease can be treated or controlled and some cannot. The more risk factors you have, and the higher their level, the greater your risk of developing coronary heart disease. Risk factors are divided into two categories:

Uncontrollable Risk Factors
(Factors we cannot modify)

Increasing Age
- Men ages 45 and older have increased risk.
- Women ages 55 and older have increased risk.

Family History
- Children of parents who developed coronary heart disease before age 55 are more likely to develop it themselves.

Racial or Ethnic Background
- African Americans, Mexican Americans, American Indians, and other Native Americans have greater risk than Caucasians.

Controllable *Risk Factors*
(Factors we can change)

- Physical Inactivity
- Smoking
- Overweight or Obesity
- High Blood Pressure
- High Blood Cholesterol
- High Blood Triglyceride
- Diabetes Mellitus
- Stress
- Hormone Replacement Therapy (HRT)

(for treatment of Menopause)

The best way to prevent coronary heart disease is to:

- Understand your risk factors
- Discuss your risk factors with your primary care physician
- Take appropriate steps to reduce your risk by …

Getting Back to BASICS.

The BASICS For Staying Healthy

It's early Saturday morning and you're lying in bed enjoying the fact that you don't have to get up early to go to work. You turn on the television to hear the morning news just as some health expert is telling you about contaminated drinking water in your neighborhood. You're fed up, you change the channel, and just in time to hear another so called expert say, *'take this medication, and you'll increase your risk of stroke and heart attack by 25 percent.'* Your wife says, give me the clicker honey - let me try. Next stop, an infomercial touting the benefits of some product guaranteed to make you lose 30 pounds in just one week. Another click and, *'call this psychic immediately to find out what you're really thinking, and best of all, what's in store for you in matters of life, health and romance.'* Your wife looks at you - you look at her - a smile comes to each of your faces and at that moment you both decide to roll over and get some more sleep. Sounds familiar? - I thought so!

Almost any day when you turn on the television, you may hear a news story about how a particular product caused some health problem. Sometimes, it gets so bad you just want to curl up under the covers and spend the day in bed. It almost seems that the path we walk in life is a minefield littered with risk factors ready to blow up in our faces. Some of us become so desensitized to these gloom and doom messages that we pay little attention to them. Still others listen to these messages and become so paranoid that they're afraid to do anything, becoming chronic procrastinators. Finally, there are those reasonable people like myself, and hopefully you, who listen to these messages and use the information to decide for themselves, what works best for them - and what doesn't.

'Life is too short to spend all of your time worrying about potential risk factors. You have to maintain a sensible approach to life which allows you to function normally, yet still be able to determine which of the numerous health advisories are important to you and which are not.'

Each of us travels down the same path of life and frequently makes decisions, which impact our lives. Occasionally, we stray from the main road by making poor health choices. If we're lucky, we soon realize our mistake, make the necessary correction, and resume our walk down the correct healthful path. Sometimes, we don't realize our mistake and travel down a path, which results in declining health. The further we walk down this path, the closer we get to the end - <u>*a dead end!*</u>

We all have choices in life. When we make good, healthful choices, we usually experience good health. When we make poor choices, we generally experience ill health. The fact is - you, not me, not anyone else, make your choices. *'Good or bad, right or wrong, <u>they're yours to make.</u>'*

It's interesting to note that millions of Americans believe that they are healthy, in spite of the fact that they are continually breaking the **BASIC** **Laws of Health** on a daily basis. Then one day out of the blue they suddenly get sick and ask themselves - why has this happened to me? In ancient days people who became sick thought they were cursed. If someone wished them ill, '*poof*', they became sick. Today, we no longer have the luxury of believing in witches, spells and curses. Yet, people still believe that someone or something else causes illness and disease. Occasionally it is, however, most often illness and disease is not caused by the curse of someone else, but rather, by the curse we bring upon ourselves. That curse being our neglect of the greatest piece of machinery ever invented, our own bodies.

I mentioned a moment ago that most of us break the Laws of Health regularly. The fact is – many of us do so without even realizing our mistakes. Still others recognizing the errors of our way continue to break the Laws of Health with no remorse. As youngsters we grew up with a sense of immortality, often performing daredevil feats we would never think of doing at this stage in our lives. In spite of the maturation process, which taught us not to behave like daredevil, Evel Knievel, we continue to break the Laws of Health with impunity. Whether we attempt to jump the Grand Canyon in a rocket cycle, or overindulge, over-excess ourselves to the extreme, the results will eventually be the same. You might fool others into thinking everything is okay. You might even fool yourself into believing it, but, if you live outside the Laws of Health, you can't fool your body. Eventually you will pay the price, that being, the premature onset of illness and disease.

Many of us recognize that we are breaking the Laws of Health, yet justify our actions because of the lifestyle we live. We rationalize that the stresses of work, home-life and relationships leave us little or no time to think about and address our personal needs. We eat poorly, sleep erratically and exercise infrequently, yet, when we get sick, someone or something else caused it. We justify our failure to live according to the Laws of Health because of too little time, overwork, over-stress, financial worries, relationship problems, child-rearing problems - the list goes on. While these factors most definitely impact on our lives and our health - the difference between whether or not we maintain good health or begin the cycle of declining health will be determined by how we identify and properly address these personal issues.

For many of us, the excuse, '*I'm too busy*' is near the top of the list of why we don't take care of ourselves. It's a convenient, believable excuse. However, it's interesting to note that when most of us are on vacation, and have a little extra time, we still eat poorly, sleep erratically and exercise infrequently. Each of us handles the challenges of life and manages our time in a different way. For some of us, procrastination is a way of life. We might have plenty of time, yet accomplish very little. I remember being told by a business colleague; when you need to get an urgent job done, give it to a busy person. He believed that the busy person, although swamped with work, was more efficient, more productive and ultimately would find a way to accomplish the task, whereas the lazy person would always find a way to procrastinate.

For some people, staying healthy seems to be easy. They can abuse their body seemingly to excess without suffering any ill consequences. It almost appears as if they have some miracle gene that makes them immune to illness and disease. They smoke, drink, overeat, and when they go for a checkup their Doctor says, *'Whatever you're doing, keep it up.'* How could that be? How is it possible to violate the Laws of Health without suffering the consequences?

The fact is – some of us have better genes than others. If you think of your genetic makeup as a series of cards shuffled in a card game, you begin to realize that, at the moment of conception, <u>some of us were dealt a better hand</u>. So what are the odds of you being dealt a genetic royal straight flush? Pretty slim, but don't feel bad. Chances are you're just like the overwhelming majority of us. You know people with blemishes and not perfect bodies, a little high blood pressure and heart disease in the family history. Factors which echo the glaring truth that, *'staying healthy just doesn't happen - but rather is the result of our personal commitment to make healthy choices.'*

It's interesting to note that, one can violate the civil or criminal laws of this country, and in some cases escape punishment. There are thousands of laws that we have created to govern our lives. So many in fact that it's quite possible to violate a law without even realizing it. However, a much higher authority designed the laws, which govern our health. These laws are part of the natural laws of the universe, and to abuse them, usually carry much stricter penalties, with offenders seldom going unpunished.

So what are the <u>BASIC Laws of Health?</u>

You Already Know Them...

- Eat Healthy Foods
- Exercise Regularly
- Drink Plenty of Water
- Get Plenty of Sleep
- Think Positively

If you follow the BASIC Laws of Health, you will turn back your biological clock and do more good for your health and well being, than might ever be done by most health practitioners or over-the-counter medications.

How Old Are You Really?

Have you ever wondered why some people age differently than others? I'll bet you have friends or relatives who look a lot older or younger than they really are. That's because we all have two ages. The first, our <u>chronological age</u> represents the number of candles we put on our birthday cake if we're being completely honest. The second, our <u>biological age</u>, often called our True Age or Real Age represents our physiologic and mental age, based on how we take care of ourselves.

It's interesting to note that many people believe that once they reach a certain age their bodies will start to deteriorate by planned obsolescence. It's almost as if they accept this decline in their health as an inevitable fact of life. But that's not the way it is. Today, it's widely accepted that if you live a healthy lifestyle you can reduce your biological age by up to 20 years.

As Research Physiologist for the Health Risk Assessment Corporation, I developed the algorithms and BioAge calculations for the TruAge computer program. This complex software calculates biological age based on the results of sophisticated physiologic tests. I've spent years statistically evaluating the influence of risk factors on biological age. Based on this research, I have no doubt that you can turn back your biological clock; improve the quality of your life and perhaps the quantity of your life if you make healthy lifestyle choices.

I bet you're thinking to yourself right now, I've been eating wrong and not exercising for twenty years, what chance do I have to turn back my biological clock? The answer is simply - it's almost never too late. The decline of one's health is not an inevitable fact of life, rather, a state of mind. Over the past twenty-five years, I have repeatedly witnessed 60-year-old men and women turn back their biological clocks and enjoy life as biological 45-year-old's.

About now, you're probably wondering, what is my biological age? While the answer to this question would be most accurately measured under laboratory conditions using sophisticated testing devices, there are some simplified tests you can perform at home. The **True Age Test** (*www.MyTrueAge.com*) was designed to give you some indication of your current biological age.

The True Age Test has two components. The first is a series of physical performance tests designed to measure several health and fitness performance parameters. **Before you attempt any of the physical performance tests - if you have any concerns about your ability to safely perform the test, do not take the test and consult with your doctor.** The second test component is a personal profile questionnaire that examines health history data and some personal lifestyle choices. <u>Please remember</u>: The True Age test is a simplified home version of a more sophisticated laboratory test to approximate your biological age. It was designed to help you identify risk factors and make appropriate lifestyle recommendations.

Your True Age Test results are a starting point. Even if your test results were positive, you have to continue to make healthy choices. If, however, your results were not what you expected, then you must carefully examine which areas of your lifestyle can be changed and do something about them. As you make positive lifestyle adjustments, over a period of time, you will significantly influence the results of future tests.

While many people are quick to offer advice on almost any topic, nobody knows you better than yourself. You have to make your own decisions in life. Those decisions will in part determine the outcome of your quest to get healthy and stay healthy. We live in a complicated world and are constantly being exposed to dangerous risk factors in the water we drink, the air we breathe, the foods we eat, and so on. In a sense, life today is risky business. As you travel the path of life each decision you make will alter your direction and possibly your health. You must constantly monitor the choices you make, to determine if they are right for you - healthy for you

Research has shown, if you quit smoking, moderate your intake of alcohol, eat healthier foods, get plenty of sleep, control stress, keep well hydrated and exercise regularly, you will turn back your biological clock. Will you live forever? of course not. However, by learning how to <u>Get Back to BASICS</u> – *'you give yourself the very best chance to enjoy a full, productive, happy, healthy and possibly - longer life.'*

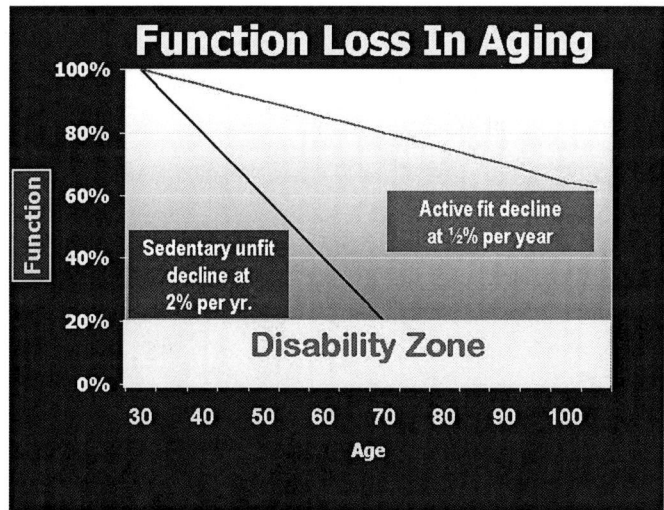

The above graph depicts <u>Functional Loss In Aging</u>. As we age, each year we lose some of our ability to perform activities of daily life. Some of us experience functional loss at a much faster rate, because of our unhealthy lifestyle. After age thirty, a sedentary (*inactive*) person (*who does not follow the Basic laws of Health*) may experience a functional decline at a rate of 2% each year, while his physically active (*health conscious*) counterpart may experience only a ½% decline yearly. By age 60 the difference is quite striking. While the physically active person may be enjoying life functioning at 85%, their unfit counterpart may functioning at 40% and headed towards partial or full disability.

The time has come for you to stop making excuses for not taking care of yourself. Now is the time to take responsibility for your health. The changes you make will improve the quality of your life – *and may save your life*.

Now is the time to rearrange your priorities and place your health and well-being at the top of the list.

If you won't do it because I tell you to, then do it for the people who really matter in your life.

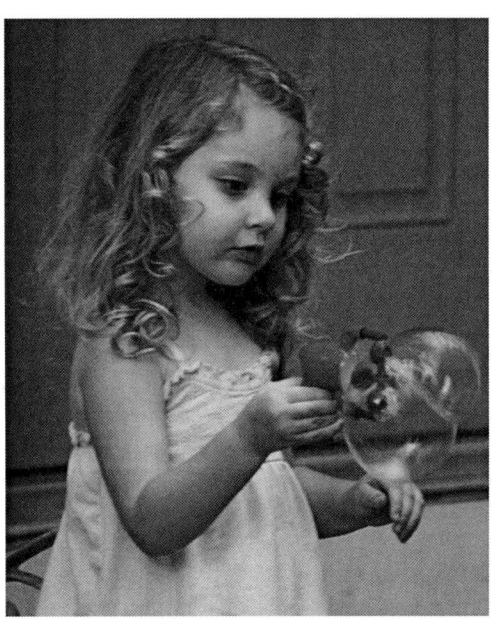
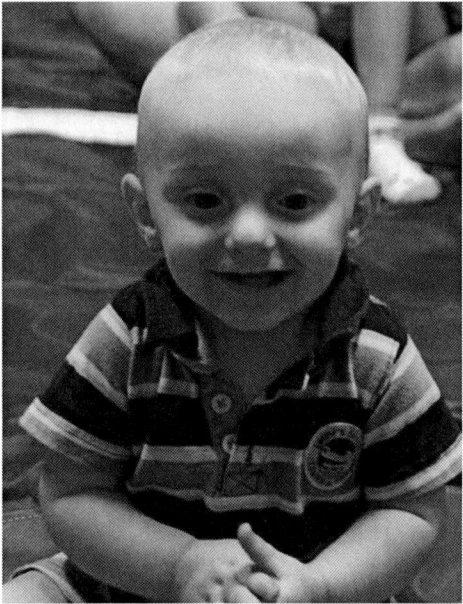

'Motivation is what gets you started...
Habit is what keeps you going'
Jim Ryan

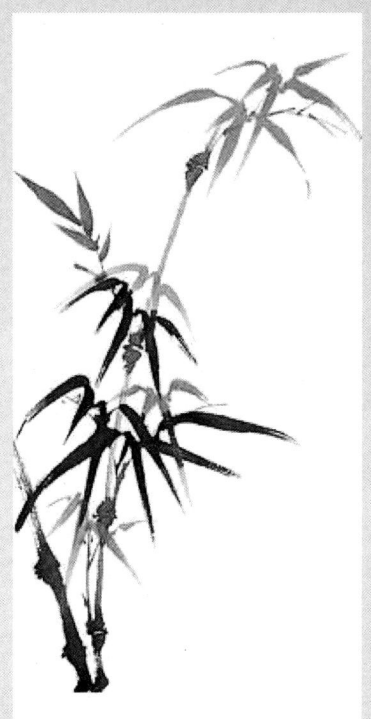

Part 3

The Weight Management Dilemma

The Obesity Epidemic

Eat Right To Stay Healthy

Some Food For Thought

Staying Fit and Healthy is a Family Responsibility

According to the U.S. Department of Health and Human Services the rate of obesity among American children has tripled since 1980. Furthermore, research has shown that from age 13 to 18, there is a steady decline in adolescent fitness. The American Council on Exercise (ACE) reports that by the time teenagers reach high school age almost 63% are physically inactive. Along with this drastic rise in childhood obesity, medical professionals have seen an alarming increase of adult medical problems (*i.e. Type II Diabetes*) developing in young children. If that's not bad enough, it's been estimated that nearly 3,000 young teenagers become new smokers every day.

As Parents we have an obligation to be positive role models for our children. If we are physically inactive, smoke and eat poorly our children are destined to follow this unhealthy example. By living a healthy lifestyle, we set a good example that will provide children with life-long wellness benefits. It's never too early to begin setting a good example.

Get Fit For Life, LLC is pleased to offer several free downloads to help parents combat childhood obesity at our www.MyTrueAge.com website.

- **'Let's Do It' - Parent/Child Incentive Program**

The Let's Do It program was designed to help parents set realistic healthy lifestyle goals for young children. The program encourages children to increase their daily activity, decrease inactive behavior and make healthy eating, drinking and snacking choices. This Let's Do It program was developed by Barry M. Stein in cooperation with The Center for Weight Management - North Shore Long Island Jewish Health System. *Get Fit For Life, LLC* is pleased to offer the Let's Do it program as a free download on our home page.

- **'The House I Live In' - Healthy Habits Activity/Coloring Book**

The House I Live In is a 16-page activity/coloring book used by parents, educators and medical professionals to teach children the importance of developing life-long healthy habits. The House I Live In (*authored by Barry M. Stein and illustrated by artist Bill Kresse*) is filled with fun activities designed to encourage parents and children (*or teachers and their class*) to have healthy lifestyle discussions. *Get Fit For Life, LLC* is pleased to offer The House I Live In as a free download on our home page.

The Obesity Epidemic

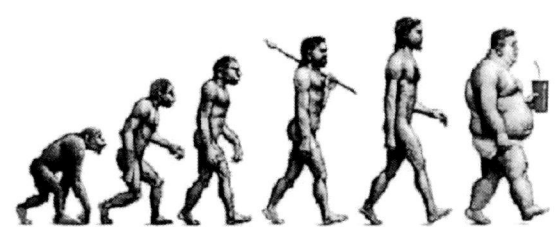

We're moving in the wrong direction

Recent statistics on the growing Obesity Epidemic have demonstrated a dangerously overweight population worldwide. Within the past 10 years, in the United States the rate of obesity has increased at a staggering rate among all groups regardless of age, gender, socio-economic level, education level and ethnicity. According to the American National Center for Health Statistics, between 1962 and 2000, the number of obese people in the US increased from 13% to an alarming 31%. Today, almost 63% of Americans are overweight (*men and women are about equally represented*) with a BMI (*body mass index*) of 25 or more.

The Challenge Of Childhood Obesity

Childhood obesity statistics reveal that one out of every three children in America has a weight problem. Even more troubling are statistics that suggest that more than 24.4% of US preschoolers are overweight - and that children who are overweight before 8 years of age, were more likely to become obese adults with their degree of obesity more severe.

During the first year of life infants normally gain weight with an increase in body fat. As a child becomes more physically active (*crawling, walking*) they tend to lose body fat. At some point a child begins to develop their adult body fat. This secondary increase in body fat is often referred to as the '*adiposity rebound.*' French researchers examining childhood obesity from infancy to school age noted that children who were able to delay the adiposity rebound past age 5, were more likely to develop a normal weight track, whereas children who experienced the rebound at a much earlier age, were more likely to become overweight children – and obese adults. The implications of this study are quite clear, '*as parents it's never too early to begin teaching children healthy habits and that if you wait until a child reaches school age – it may be too late.*'

Percentage of Overweight Children

The National Health and Nutrition Examination Survey (NHANES) study (2003-2006) highlighted the alarming trend in childhood obesity.

	Survey (1976-80)	*Survey (2003-2006)*
Age (2-5) years	5.0%	24.4%
Age (6-11) years	6.5%	33.3%
Age (12-19) years	5.0%	34.1%

As an associate in the Department of Medicine - North Shore-LIJ Health System (2003–2009), I was part of The Center for Weight Management clinical weight management team. This multi-disciplinary program dealt with the complex issues of adult and childhood obesity. This comprehensive program focused on the medical, nutritional, exercise and behavioral needs of overweight, obese and bariatric surgery patients.

In 2003, I presented at a program aptly titled, The Obesity Epidemic at the North Shore University Hospital in Manhasset, New York. At this conference, Dr. Cara Ebbeling, PhD, from the Division of Endocrinology at Children's Hospital in Boston discussed the Key Issues In Obesity Prevention. Dr. Ebbeling began by saying, *'Historically, a fat child meant a healthy child, one who was likely to survive the rigors of undernourishment and infection. However, in the past decade, excessive fatness has arguably become the primary childhood health problem in this and many other parts of the world.'*

While the causes of childhood obesity are complex (*genetics, activity, diet, family, environmental*) according to Dr. Ebbeling there are several common sense approaches to prevention and treatment that include:

Home
- Set aside time for healthy meals
- Increase physical activity
- Limit television viewing

School
- Fund mandatory physical education
- Establish strict guidelines for school lunch programs
- Establish and implement school wellness polices

Healthcare
- Improve insurance coverage for effective obesity treatment
- Provide coverage for obesity prevention

Marketing and Media
- Consider a tax on fast foods and soft drinks
- Prohibit food advertising and marketing directed at children
- Increase public funding for obesity prevention education

Politics
- Regulate political contributions from the food industry

It's widely known that bodyweight is regulated by numerous physiologic mechanisms that maintain balance between energy intake (*calories in*) and energy expenditure (*calories out*). Under normal conditions these regulatory systems are extraordinarily precise. However, it only takes a positive energy balance of 120 calories daily (*one sugar-sweetened soft drink*) above your body's normal daily caloric requirement, to produce a weight increase of 12 lbs each year. Multiply that by ten years – and you have … *morbid obesity*.

How can you tell if you're at a healthy weight?

Calculate Your BMI

One way to determine whether your weight is healthy for you is to calculate your body mass index *(BMI)* which measures the relationship between your height and weight. The Centers for Disease Control website offers free adult and child BMI calculators at: http://www.cdc.gov/healthyweight/assessing/bmi/index.html

ADULT - BMI results

BMI (less than 18.5)   - *underweight*
BMI (18.5 to 24.9)   - *normal or healthy weight*
BMI (25.0 to 29.9)   - *overweight*
BMI (30.0 or higher)   - *obese*

Another way to determine if you are overweight is to calculate your waist circumference. Excessive abdominal fat in adults is serious, because it increases your risk for developing obesity-related disorders, such as Type II Diabetes, high blood cholesterol, elevated triglycerides, high blood pressure, and coronary artery disease. Your waistline may be telling you that you're at risk if you are:

- A man whose waist circumference is more than 40 inches

- A non-pregnant woman whose waist circumference is more than 35 inches

CHILD - BMI results

To determine whether your child is at a healthy weight, calculate their body mass index *(BMI)* using the child BMI calculator on The Centers for Disease Control website. Based on their BMI percentile (*separate for boys and girls*) your child will fall into one of 4 categories:

    Below 5th percentile   – ***underweight***
    $5^{th} - 84^{th}$ percentile   – ***normal or healthy weight***
    $85^{th} - 94^{th}$ percentile   – ***overweight***
    Above 95th percentile   – ***obese***

Listed below are some valuable weight management websites that provide free information and programming targeting adult and childhood obesity.

Adult / Childhood Obesity Resources

http://www.MyTrueAge.com
An online health and wellness resource for individuals and families seeking services, information and products pertaining to adult and childhood weight management. This site offers a free parent-child weight management program entitled; *Let's Do It,* a free children's healthy habits activity/coloring book, *The House I Live In*. - and a free online *True Age Test* - to find out how old you really are.

http://win.niddk.nih.gov/
Weight Control Information Network, an information service of the National Institutes of Health and National Institute of Diabetes and Digestive and Kidney Diseases. WIN provides the general public, health professionals, the media, and Congress with up-to-date, science-based information on weight control, obesity, physical activity, and related nutritional issues.

http://www.shapeup.org
Shape Up America! is a 501(c)3 not-for-profit organization committed to raising awareness of obesity as a health issue. The mission of Shape Up America! is to provide evidence-based information and guidance on weight management to the public, health care professionals, educators, policymakers and the media.

www.diabetes.org
Website of the American Diabetes Association, the nation's leading nonprofit health organization providing diabetes research, information and advocacy. Look here for science-based information about diabetes related nutrition topics, recipes, exercise tips and the latest research. Plus - find out what's happening locally in your community.

www.eatright.org
Website of the American Dietetic Association, the best source for sound nutritional guidance in the US.

Eat Right To Stay Healthy

By now you know that over 60% of all Americans are overweight? And approximately a third would be considered obese? Many medical experts agree that obesity may be the greatest health risk confronting Americans today. While many factors influence our general health, by far, the most important is our diet. Yet, for many of us, our entire existence seems to revolve around mealtime. We forget that the primary objective of eating is to supply our bodies with the nutrients essential for life. Instead, we over-eat foods of questionable nutritional value because they taste good. In other words, we don't care whether a particular food is good for us, as long as it pleases our taste buds. For many of us, our unhealthy philosophy of eating may be summed up as, *Live To Eat*, instead of the more sensible, healthful approach, <u>Eat To Live</u>.

It appears that many of us consider eating almost a religious experience. From the moment we awake in the morning, until retiring at night, we plan our whole day thinking of new and unusual ways to please our taste buds. Our whole psyche is wrapped up in the eating experience and the pleasure we derive from it.

In this country there are laws against committing suicide. However, there are no laws against eating yourself to death. Yet, each year millions of Americans do just that. Unfortunately, there are no laws against gluttony. If there were, we could probably save countless lives. The unhealthy philosophy of *Live To Eat* will likely be the number one reason why so many of us will not be able to fully enjoy our retirement years. If your life revolves around over-eating unhealthy foods, you are destined to suffer the unpleasant consequences.

Eating right means making the decision to eat foods, which promote good health. That doesn't mean that you can't cheat on occasion. Sometimes it's good for the psyche to cheat a little. The problem arises when cheating becomes the rule, rather than the exception. Rewarding oneself at the end of the day by eating a whole box of *Oreo's* is not sensible eating. You have to take responsibility for your actions. Nobody is going to force-feed you those *Oreo's*. If you know that you're the type of person that can't eat just one or two, then don't buy them.

I recently had a conversation with a new patient who complained that, although she was exercising regularly, she wasn't losing any weight. I asked her about her dietary habits and was not surprised with her response. While she generally ate good foods, she made some basic eating mistakes, which made her desired weight loss goal almost impossible to achieve.

> '*What would you consider to be your biggest dietary mistake?*' I asked.
>
> '*Well, I sort of have a thing for blueberry pie and ice cream.*'

'How often do you indulge yourself?'

'I have a piece of pie and a dish of ice cream almost every night.'

'You have a piece of blueberry pie and ice cream almost every night?'

'I hate to waste any of the pie so I have a piece every night until I finish it.'

'And you put ice cream on the pie as well?' I added.

'No, I have the ice cream separately.'

'You mean you have a piece of pie and dish of ice cream every night?'

'That's right.'

'Don't you think that this would have a bearing on whether or not you are able to lose weight?'

'Oh, I know it does - but I can't help myself - I still do it. If there's a piece of pie left, I'll eat it.'

'Have you ever thought about not buying pie or ice cream?'

'Yes, many times - but I still do it. I'm angry with myself because I'm usually quite disciplined in other areas of my life.'

'Remember, I mentioned to you that it's 'okay' to eat sweets on occasion?'

'Yes, I remember you saying that.'

'Do you remember that I said it should be on occasion and not all the time?'

'I remember, but once I buy the pie I feel obligated to finish it.'

'Have you ever though about cutting the pie into small portions and freezing them?'

'No.'

'What if I told you it would be all right to have two portions each week?'

'I guess I could try that.'

'You know, one of the biggest challenges of eating properly is that we are always trying to please our palate, our taste buds. If pie and ice cream are available we generally will chose it, instead of a healthy snack.'

'So you're saying that if it's available around the house, I'll eat it?'

'Absolutely. For most of us, there is no choice between a piece of cake or a carrot. Once you buy that blueberry pie and ice cream, you feel obligated to eat it. The key word to remember is <u>availability</u>. If it's available, you'll eat it.'

'So you're saying don't buy it?'

'That would be a good idea. However, if you must, then you have to find a way to regulate your eating style so that you eat it occasionally - rather than all the time.'

This conversation is a clear example of how food can be used as a daily reward in our unhealthy quest to please our taste buds. By catering to food cravings, we make a serious eating mistake, which may prevent us from achieving our weight goal and better health.

I once asked a class of college students the difference between the words <u>appetite</u> and <u>hunger</u>. Surprisingly, more than 50% of the class replied there was no difference. I then asked; if you were marooned on a desert island what foods would you miss the most? Not surprisingly, almost 75% of the class responded naming junk foods containing a ton of calories with minimal nutritional value. All I can say is, radio and television advertisers have done an admirable job teaching intelligent people how to eat poorly.

<u>Consider the following</u>: If an advertising company were touting the benefits of smoking cigarettes on Sunday morning television, the public outcry would be deafening. Government agencies would immediately step in to punish the perpetrators of this heinous crime. Yet each day, a new crop of youngsters is subtly influenced by media advertisements, to believe that many nutritionally valueless foods are good to eat. While this may seem irresponsible, bordering on criminal, I can still remember bugging my parents, forty-eight years ago, to buy a particular brand of breakfast cereal so that I could get the prize in the box.

So, what's the difference between appetite and hunger? Appetite is the craving you get for foods you like to eat, even if you're not hungry. Hunger is the feeling you get when your body needs fuel. If you were on a desert island with an abundance of natural foods (*fish, fruit, berries*), you might get a craving for an unavailable cheeseburger - that would be appetite. On the other hand, if there were no readily available food sources and you were slowly starving to death, you would forage for anything to stay alive - that would be hunger. In a sense, appetite is a mental thing, a craving, whereas hunger is a physiological thing. While it's quite possible that a person could die from hunger and starvation – <u>no one ever dies from appetite cravings</u>.

A secondary, yet equally important eating issue, has to do with the amount of food we eat - portion size. Many of us have been brought up to believe, *'if it's on the plate - you have to eat it.'* To this day, I can remember my own mother encouraging me to finish everything on my plate, because there were people starving in other countries.

During the mid-1970's, I directed the Laboratory of Applied Physiology at the Cardiac Rehabilitation Center in Miami. Many of the cardiac patients I worked with made restaurant recommendations, often saying, *'the early bird special was excellent and best of all, it was - all you can eat.'* Almost as if all you can eat was a selling point. Here was a group of serious cardiac patients that needed to carefully watch what they ate and how much they ate - telling me where to get the best - all you can eat buffet.'

At this point in our lives, we have to remember that the amount we eat *(portion size)* is as important as what we eat. If you're looking to lose weight, reducing portion size is the sensible way to reach your goal. Contrary to what you may have been told, there is no mystery to weight gain and weight loss. If you think of your weight like a bank balance, if you put in more dollars (*calories*) your balance (*weight*) - goes up. As you withdraw funds (*eat fewer calories*) your balance (*weight*) - goes down. If you eat fewer calories and exercise regularly, you'll lose weight even faster.

Albert J. Bellows, M.D. in his book, The Philosophy of Eating, wrote, *'If science in farming is important, as it has proven to be, may not science in eating be more important?'* Dr. Bellows suggests, that while scientists may have made every conceivable effort to increase their knowledge of how best to grow food, people still haven't learned how to eat right. Dr. Bellows published, The Philosophy of Eating in the year 1870. Here was a 139 year-old diet book stating that people back then didn't eat right.

If Dr. Bellows was correct, that our ancestors ate poorly 139 years ago, think about life today. Back then people ate natural, unprocessed foods. There were no pesticides, chemically treated foods, artificial flavors - no junk foods. In comparison today, virtually everything we put in our mouths has been altered in some way.

Our lives today are very different than our ancestors living 100 years ago. Most days are filled with so many things to do and problems to solve, that we seldom take the time to eat properly. Our so-called *'civilized culture'* presents us with so many life challenges that we are often pressured to make unhealthy eating choices. It's difficult to rush meals during the day and still select healthy foods. For many of us, candy bars and junk foods are a principal part of our regular diet.

The appetite center in our brain constantly sends us subconscious messages throughout the day. The message we perceive may tell us that we're thirsty, crave a particular food, or we're truly hungry. Sometimes the appetite center sends us a message to, '*Eat that chocolate donut, or else.*' So what do we generally do? - we eat that donut. Once the craving is satisfied and our taste buds have been appeased, the appetite center shuts down and we feel better.

When we're really hungry, our appetite center sends us a completely different message, '*we're running on empty so FILL'ER UP!*' At times like these, if we eat fast, we generally will eat too much. That's because it takes approximately 15 minutes for the appetite center in your brain to stop sending '*I'm hungry messages*' after it began telling you to eat. Most of us can do a lot of caloric damage in 15 minutes.

One surprisingly easy way to gain control over '*I'm hungry*' messages is to slow down your eating speed. To accomplish this simply chew each bite of food 12-24 times before swallowing. The slower you eat, the easier it will be for you to reduce the amount you eat. If you can delay your meal past the 15-minute mark, those unpleasant feelings of hunger will be gone, and you won't eat as much. Chewing foods 12-24 times will not only slow down your eating speed, but it will also help solve another serious eating problem.

When you eat fast you don't chew foods properly. Chewing is a part of the normal digestive process that breaks foods down into smaller pieces. By eating fast, you bypass this important mechanical process leaving more work for the stomach. Your stomach will make a valiant effort to complete the food breakdown process, but if it has a problem, you'll know it when you get an upset stomach. If you think of your digestive system as an assembly line, if the guys at the front of the line are not doing their job, this creates problems further down the line.

In 1913, Horace Fletcher published an interesting book entitled, *FLETCHERISM: What It Is*. Surprisingly, this 223-page book described in detail how one should chew their foods properly in order to stay healthy. It's hard to believe that someone could actually write 223 pages on the topic of chewing. Besides that, it's not everyday that you get to read a book that has a chapter titled, '*How To Masticate Properly.*' Calm down folks - the word was masticate, as in chew your foods. What could you possibly be thinking? Fletcher's eating philosophy became quite popular at that time and was known as Fletcherism. His disciples were called Fletcherites. Counted among his followers was John D. Rockerfeller, perhaps the wealthiest financier of his day. In Horace Fletchers own words, Fletcherism was based on the idea that:

'I chew my foods carefully until I extract all taste from it ... and until it slipped unconsciously down my throat. When the appetite ceased, and I was thereby told that I had had enough, I stopped; and I had no desire to eat any more until a real appetite commanded me again. Then I again chewed carefully.'

I believe that our cultural eating habits today are the direct opposite of what Horace Fletcher proposed 96 years ago. Instead of savoring the texture and flavor of foods by chewing foods carefully, more than likely we gulp foods, because we don't have the time to eat slowly. Today there are no Fletcherites around. If there were, I am sure that they would be appalled by the way we eat. I can still remember, years ago as a child, my mother admonishing me to, be home at 6 o'clock for dinner or else. Heaven help me if I was late for dinner, with or without a good excuse. Mealtime in our family was an unhurried family get-together. We talked about the events of the day and my parents always cautioned me to eat slowly and chew my food carefully. Sounds like they might have been Fletcherites. Today, most families rarely sit down for a leisurely meal together.

Because of our complex lifestyle, many of us are often forced to skip meals and may end up snacking all day. Your digestive system can handle three, four, possibly five feedings a day, however, any more than that places undo strain on the system. Just as your muscles need both exercise and rest, your digestive system also needs some down time.

I generally advise people to:

Eat A Good Breakfast

Try To Have Your **Big Meal** In The Afternoon

Eat A Light Dinner

And Little Or Nothing After 8 P.M.

I call a good breakfast *'FOOD FOR FUEL.'* Breakfast gets you going as you become physically active at the start of your day. I call a late meal, *'FOOD FOR FAT.'* In the evening, our basal metabolic rate is slowing down as we become less physically active. Why fill up your stomach with food when your body doesn't need it?

Clients often tell me that they skip eating breakfast because they're not hungry in the morning. The logic they employ to come to that decision almost makes sense. That being, *'if they don't feel hungry and they want to lose weight - they shouldn't eat.'* Before you start skipping breakfast you should know that your mother was right when she said breakfast is the most important meal of the day. Although you may not feel hungry in the morning, under normal conditions your blood sugar level will generally be low. If you don't eat breakfast, as the morning progresses, your blood sugar level will continue to drop. By the time lunch arrives, it may be so low that you'll eat anything that's not nailed down. By eating a balanced breakfast, you help your body to regulate your blood sugar level so that you don't rebound between sugar highs and lows. <u>In the long run eating a light breakfast will help you to lose weight</u>.

While we're on the topic of blood sugar levels, let's take a moment to talk about processed sugar. Historically, 100 years ago the average American consumed about 5-pounds of sugar each year. If you imagine a 5-pound sack of sugar you would probably think that this was an unusually large amount. In comparison, the average American today may consume more than 10 times that amount. Is it any wonder that obesity and diabetes are so prevalent among Americans? I once watched as a friend of mine spooned eight teaspoons of sugar into a cup of coffee. It seemed to me that there was more sugar in that cup than coffee. The fact that our taste buds have become so accustomed to sweets makes it difficult for us to avoid them. The time has come for us to reeducate our taste buds to accept foods that are not saturated with sugar.

While we're on the topic of sugar, I feel compelled to say a few words about sugar substitutes. While sugar substitutes don't pile up the calories, they also don't allow you to make that all-important palate change. If you're hooked on sweets and use artificial sweeteners as a substitute, your taste buds can't distinguish between what's real and what's not. If you don't train your taste buds not to crave sweets, they will keep prodding you to eat them whether they're real or artificial. One additional thing to consider is that some people, without realizing it, are allergic to aspartame, a commonly used sugar substitute.

Let's take a moment to talk about salt. It's widely known that excess dietary salt causes retention of fluids, which ultimately may raise your blood pressure. If your diet consists of snacks like pretzels, potato chips, and you frequently add salt to foods, you're overdoing it Foods heavily laden with salt should be placed on the occasional list, not the every day snack food list.

While I don't recommend vegetarianism for everyone, I do believe that it is a good idea to significantly reduce the amount of animal fat, particularly red meat, in your diet. There is an overwhelming amount of evidence which links elevated blood cholesterol levels to a significantly increased risk of high blood pressure, heart attack and stroke. For many years it's been widely known that these excess blood fats deposit themselves on the inside walls (*lumen*) of arteries. As this occurs, the diameter of the artery gets smaller, and more pressure is needed to pump blood through these partially clogged blood vessels. At some point, if they become totally clogged - <u>you have a big problem</u>.

By now you must realize that my message to you is clear. Eating should not be viewed as a religious experience; it's a function of life. Eat right and you have a better chance to stay healthy. Eat wrong and you will suffer the consequences. Now is the time to stop pleasing your taste buds and begin to focus on eating foods that are good for you. Don't let yourself become fooled into thinking that since you feel all right, everything must be just fine. It's well documented that <u>heart attacks and strokes are culminating events that follow years of personal neglect</u>. Now is the time to begin taking control of your life and make healthy eating choices.

Let's summarize some important points of this chapter

- The primary objective of eating is to supply our bodies with the nutrients essential for life.

- Don't <u>LIVE TO EAT</u>. Learn to <u>EAT TO LIVE</u>.

- As I mentioned in the blueberry pie story at the beginning of this chapter <u>availability</u> is the key word. If it's available, <u>you'll eat it</u>.

- Eat slowly and chew each bite of food at least 12-24 times before swallowing. Don't rush meals. Take your time and <u>savor the flavor</u>.

- Eat a good breakfast - <u>Food For Fuel</u>.

- Don't eat after 8 p.m. - <u>Food For Fat</u>.

- Sugar and Salt should be used moderately - if at all.

- You don't have to finish everything on the plate.

- Eat right and you have a better chance to stay healthy. Eat wrong and you will suffer the consequences.

Some FOOD for THOUGHT

While I'm not a Registered Dietician, over the years I have had the opportunity to work with many nutrition experts. At the Cardiac Rehabilitation Center in Miami patients stayed with us for 28 days. They ate foods prepared by special chefs and received instruction in how to purchase and prepare foods. The following eating suggestions are a conglomeration of meal plan ideas I received from different sources over the past twenty-five years. I stress the word <u>suggestions</u>, since you must decide if they make sense for you.

If you're overweight, these dietary suggestions will help you to lose weight. <u>Remember</u>: even if you lose a half-pound every week, you'll eventually reach your desired weight goal.

Before I begin to describe my eating suggestions, I want you to know that, in spite of what you think or may have been told, <u>it's never too late to begin eating healthy foods</u>. Occasionally, people tell me that they expected to gain weight because they reached a certain age. If that were true, everyone at the same age should be fat. The reality is, as we get older and retire from work many of us become physically inactive and have more time to eat.

As I mentioned before, there's no mystery to weight gain and weight loss. If you think of your weight as a bank balance, when you put in more dollars (*calories*) your balance (*weight*) <u>goes up</u>. As you withdraw funds (*eat fewer calories*), your balance (*weight*) <u>goes down</u>. If you <u>eat fewer calories and exercise</u>, you'll lose weight even faster and will probably keep it off.

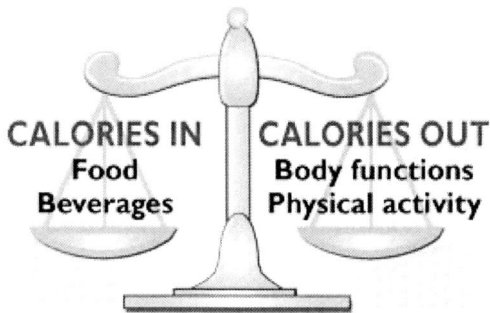

The next three pages will present several meal suggestions for your consideration. While these suggestions have been valuable for many,

<u>*You must decide whether or not they make sense for you.*</u>

BREAKFAST SUGGESTIONS

Breakfast is probably the most important meal of the day. It provides you with FOOD FOR FUEL.

DAY 1
1 egg (*use cooking spray - no butter/margarine/oil*)
1 slice of low calorie - whole wheat bread
1 fruit (*refer to fruit list*)
Coffee/herb tea (*preferably decaf*)

DAY 2
1 serving breakfast cereal (*low or no fat/sugar*)
Skim or 1% milk for cereal
1 fruit (*refer to fruit list*)
Coffee/herb tea (*preferably decaf*)

DAY 3
1 slice of low calorie - whole wheat bread
Top with low fat - cottage cheese
1 fruit (*refer to fruit list*)
Coffee/herb tea (*preferably decaf*)

FRUIT LIST
½ grapefruit
½ cantaloupe
1-cup strawberries
1-cup raspberries
1 apple
1 orange
1 peach
1 tangerine

LUNCH SUGGESTIONS

Whenever possible, I recommend that you eat your big meal of the day during the afternoon.

Main Entree
(Choice of)

(4) oz. turkey breast
(4) oz. chicken breast
1-can tuna in water
(4) oz. fresh fish
1-cup plain yogurt

Side dishes
(Choice of)

Salad (*use balsamic vinegar for dressing, no oil, no prepared dressing*)
2 vegetables (*refer to vegetable list*)
1 fruit (*refer to fruit list*)
1 cup of brown rice

VEGETABLE LIST
(*Vegetables may be eaten raw or steamed 5 minutes*)

Lettuce	Cauliflower
Tomatoes	Squash
Mushrooms	Cucumber
Radishes	Cabbage
Spinach	String beans
Red/Green Peppers	Celery
Snow Peas	Asparagus

DINNER SUGGESTIONS

Dinner is a dangerous meal for most of us. After a hard day, we tend to overeat at this meal. Remember to chew each bite of food at least 12-24 times. The slower you eat, the more likely you will turn off the appetite center and stop those unpleasant feelings of hunger. This will allow you to eat less and may help you to lose weight.

Main Entree
(Choice of)

(4-6) oz. turkey breast
(4-6) oz. chicken breast
(4-6) oz. fresh fish

(Below limited to 2 servings per week)
(4-6) oz. red meat (*roast beef, steak, pot roast - <u>no gravy</u>*)
(4-6) oz. meat (*veal, lamb or pork chops - <u>no gravy</u>*)

Side Dishes
(Choice of)

Salad (*use balsamic vinegar for dressing, no oil, no prepared dressing*)
2 vegetables (*refer to vegetable list*)
1 fruit (*refer to fruit list*)
1-cup of corn kernels

(Below limited to 2 servings per week)
Small baked potato with skin (*no sour cream*)
1-cup whole grain pasta (*low fat sauce*)

Between Meal Snacks
Keep plenty of cut-up vegetables available
1 extra fruit
Raw almonds (*1 ounce*)
Part-Skim string mozzarella cheese

So there you have it, some FOOD for THOUGHT. You can either take some of my suggestions, all of my suggestions, or none of my suggestions. You have to make your own decision. Just remember, everyone on planet Earth is on some form of diet. For some of us, pepperoni pizza is diet food, while for others; it's bean sprouts and alfalfa. I believe there's a middle ground that allows us to eat healthy, without having to feel nutritionally deprived. The time is now to take control of your eating and stop catering to your taste buds.

12-Tips To Help You Lose Weight

Tip 1. As Horace Fletcher would advise, don't eat unless you're hungry. Don't start stuffing your face because it's time to eat, you're having a bad day or your appetite center demands a piece of cake. The only time you should eat is when you're truly hungry. You can do it!

Tip 2. Exercise will help you lose or maintain weight, because it burns calories. If you think of your body as a furnace, when you exercise you make it run hotter. This will require it to use more fuel - calories.

Tip 3. Eat more fruits. The natural sugars they contain are good for your body. You might try adding several different fruits to your morning breakfast.

Tip 4. Eat more vegetables. I often hear people say that they don't eat vegetables. Vegetables are an essential part of a healthy diet and will help you to lose weight. Eat them raw, steamed or micro-waved.

Tip 5. Salads are great, but salad dressings may not be. It depends on what you consider to be an appropriate salad dressing. While balsamic vinegar and herbs are good, many prepared salad dressings are high in calories and fat. Other good salad toppings include: canola or olive oil and lemon juice.

Tip 6. It's a good idea to keep healthy snacks readily available. If you like carrots or celery, cut them up and keep them in a zip lock bag in the refrigerator. You might also try nonfat yogurt, fresh fruit, rice cakes, raw almonds or part-skim string mozzarella cheese.

Tip 7. Clean out your kitchen closets of cakes and candies. Walk over to your refrigerator and dump out the ice cream and sodas. You cannot buy these things and control your weight. As I told you before, availability is the key word. If it's available you'll eat it. You have to reeducate your taste buds to enjoy foods that are not drenched in sugar. This single palate change will go a long way toward making you healthier and slimmer.

Tip 8. Eat a light breakfast every day. Try mixing Quaker Oats with skim milk or low fat (1%) milk and your favorite fruits. (*Strawberries, blueberries, peaches, mangos, etc.*) You might even add some unsalted, roasted soybeans or raw almonds to make homemade granola.

Tip 9. Drink (8) glasses of WATER each day. It's important physiologically and will help you to lose weight.

Tip 10. When dining out, or '*in*' for that matter, add extra vegetables to your meal instead of extra starches. Ask for a double portion of vegetables instead of a baked potato or French fries.

Tip 11. I recommend weight management patients weigh themselves every day - but don't use the scale as your sole indicator of how you are doing. Weighing yourself every morning at the same time allows you to track the changes in your weight on a daily basis. In doing so, you become your own '*personal scientist*' allowing you to note your weight trend (*up or down*) - helping you to make better choices during the day. If you are just starting to exercise, it's possible to see a slight weight gain on the scale. That's because muscle, which is solid, weighs more than fat. If this happens, ask yourself, '*Do I feel better? Are my clothes fitting me better?*' If the answer to these questions is yes - then keep it up.

Tip 12. Drive past those Fast Food restaurants. It's impossible to lose weight and stay healthy if you continually eat unhealthy junk food. Take responsibility for your eating and learn how to prepare healthy foods at home. In the long run, it's a lot cheaper and much healthier. If you must eat out, look for restaurants that serve grilled chicken or fish and plenty of veggies.

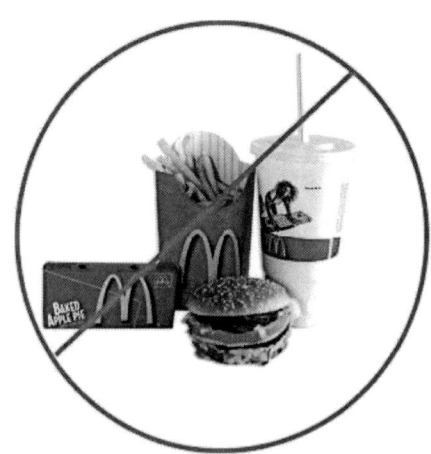

*'Effort is a commitment to seeing a task through to the end...
Not just until you get tired of it.'*
Howard Cate

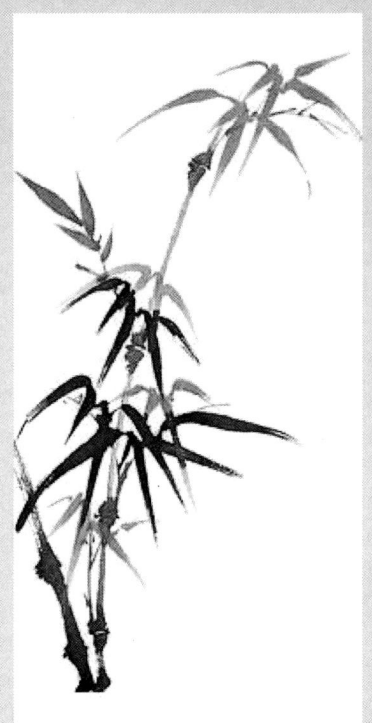

Part 4

Exercise: <u>*Essential*</u>, Not Optional

Exercise Promotes Better Health
Develop A Healthy Heart
Sensible Guidelines For Resistance Training
Keep Well Hydrated: Drink Water
Stretching May Prevent Injuries

Exercise: *Essential*, Not Optional

While it's widely known that the benefits we derive from regular exercise are essential to maintain good health, most of us still lead inactive lifestyles. For many of us, exercise is one of the last things on our *To Do List*. We know it's good for us, but we almost never find the time to do it. Today, the realities of our changing world have made it abundantly clear that regular exercise can change our lives; making us healthier, more productive and better able to meet the stressful challenges of our complex world.

To maintain your good health, and weather the current financial storm, requires a solid commitment to make healthy choices. I remember as a child being told, 'when the going gets tough … the tough get going.' Well, that time has come. The <u>going *is* tough</u> and it's time for you to - <u>*get going*</u>.

Beginning to exercise is no easy task. It requires that you make a mental adjustment, clearly prioritizing and defining what's important to you - and why. No longer can you view exercise as a choice. Instead it must become a non-negotiable part of your life. As you begin to understand that exercise is essential, not optional – you take another important step towards …

Getting Back to <u>BASICS</u>.

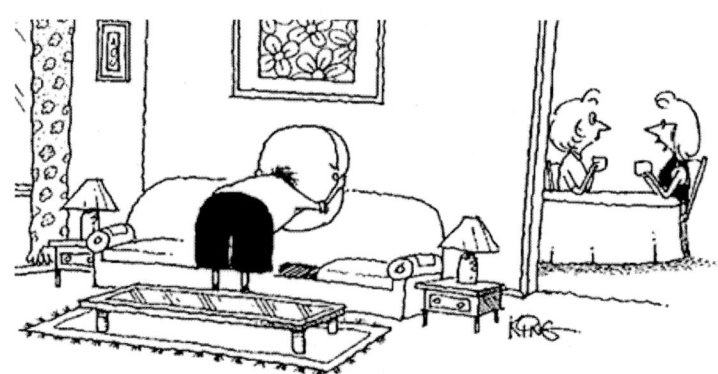

The doctor said he needed more activity. So I hide his T.V. remote three times a week.

Exercise Promotes Better Health

There is no doubt that we live in an *Age of Convenience* which has significantly reduced our need and desire to remain physically active. One hundred years ago life was very different. There were no cars, buses, airplanes, televisions, radios, computers, cellular phones, you know, all those things we count on to make our lives a little easier. We've become so dependent upon these conveniences, that when the car breaks down or the television doesn't work, it's a big deal. Our lives have become so connected to these conveniences that we find it difficult to imagine life without them.

Fifty years ago, Jack LaLanne was all alone touting the importance of regular exercise. Back then he was considered to be an exercise fanatic by many Americans. Today, he is considered to be an exercise guru. This change in the publics perception of this well-known exercise personality has occurred because we now recognize that what he was saying fifty years ago was true and remains true today:

'That one derives great health benefits from participation in a program of regularly scheduled exercise.'

The importance of regular exercise is well documented, and yet many Americans still lead inactive lives. It appears that the technological innovations over the last one hundred years, while allowing us to produce more goods and services, has created a population of people who sit behind desks for the majority of their lives, leaving them prone to the diseases of our civilized world. In a sense, as our world has changed, so have we, becoming physically inactive, over-stressed smokers who eat poorly. While the message is clear that exercise promotes good health, the reality remains that most people don't exercise regularly and that the majority of people who begin an exercise program - <u>quit</u>.

People travel many paths in their quests to become physically fit. Some join health clubs or corporate fitness programs, while others walk, jog, play golf or tennis. Unfortunately, the road to becoming physically fit is often littered with unused health club memberships and discarded fitness equipment. All too often, people stop exercising because they sustain preventable injuries or aggravate previously existing medical conditions. While most medical doctors encourage their patients to exercise, very few have the time or expertise to properly evaluate, guide and supervise exercise programs.

Currently, the majority of adult Americans do little or no exercise at all. According to a Report from the Surgeon General of the United States entitled <u>Physical Activity and Health</u>:

'That despite common knowledge that exercise is healthful, more than 60% of American adults are not regularly active and 25% of the adult population are not active at all. Moreover, although many people have enthusiastically embarked on vigorous exercise programs at one time or another, most do not sustain their participation....'

The Surgeon General warns that lack of exercise is detrimental to your health and advises at least 30 minutes of moderate exercise daily. A program of regular exercise:

- Reduces stress

- Increases self-esteem and promotes a feeling of well-being

- Reduces your risk of heart disease

- Reduces your risk of developing high blood pressure

- Reduces your risk of developing diabetes

- Promotes healthy bones, muscles and joints

- Assists in weight loss and weight control

- Helps fight depression

It's not that we don't know that we must exercise in order to remain healthy; it's just that most of us have had bad experiences when we tried. I'll bet you didn't know that statistically, more people quit health clubs than join them. Why is this, you ask? In some cases the answer may be that the club is too crowded at the time they intend to use it, or the new member feels intimidated by the surroundings. All too often, however, the main reason why a health club member stops using a club is because they hurt themselves during their first few workouts.

We've been brought up believing that in order to get physically fit you must subscribe to the notion, '*no pain - no gain.*' While this philosophy may be valid for a young athlete or body builder, it's not for a pencil-pushing, baby boomer trying to get fit after ten, twenty or thirty years of physical neglect.

You have to recognize that it took time to get out-of-shape and it will take time to get back into shape. <u>YOU CAN'T GET FIT FAST</u>! You can't rush the process without hurting yourself. If you try, you'll probably end up just another health club casualty, paying dues for a membership you don't use.

It's also interesting to note that many of us begin an exercise program for all the wrong reasons. I can't tell you how many times I've heard people say that they exercise so that they can fit into a particular dress or suit for a wedding. Invariably, whether they achieve their goal or not, once the wedding date passes, they stop exercising. You have to understand that, if you begin an exercise program with a short-term goal in mind, you're doomed to fail. One must begin an exercise program with a long-term goal in mind; to develop a pattern of regular exercise that will keep you physically fit - <u>for life</u>.

So what is an over-weight, over-stressed, pencil pusher to do when they want to get back into shape? Having assisted in writing the curriculum for the Exercise Science/Personal Training program for The City University of New York (CUNY) my suggestion is – *'If you seek the services of a professional trainer, ask about their qualifications. Do they have a degree in health and physical education, exercise physiology or certification from a professional fitness association? If not, look elsewhere.'* If you're planning to join a health club, inquire about the credentials of their staff. You don't need a pretty face and body teaching you how to get back into shape. By virtue of the fact that you're out-of-shape and maybe a few years past thirty-five, you already have some risk factors which must be addressed. Besides your age, there's a good chance that you're over-weight, have a slight blood pressure problem, just a touch of sugar in your urine and may have an abnormal EKG. You might have some of these, or all of these - and not know it. In order to be sensible, before starting any new program of exercise, <u>make an appointment for a complete medical checkup</u>.

Once the checkup is out of the way and you have the green light from your doctor, you have to make an important decision. Are you going to seek professional assistance to get started or try to do it on your own? If you intend to contract with a personal trainer or health club, make sure that the person you entrust to help you get started is sensitive to your special needs. If you intend to do it on your own, remember,

<u>Exercise is like Medicine</u>

*'While too little may not be therapeutic
<u>too much can be dangerous</u>'*

If you haven't been exercising for quite a while, you need to start out slowly. <u>As you begin an exercise program, your body needs time to gradually adjust to the increasing demands you place on it</u>. If you try to get fit fast, chances are that you will unintentionally over-stress yourself, which may result in some type of injury.

I expect that some fitness professionals might disagree with the program I am about to present. That doesn't upset me. I've learned a long time ago that, if you put five fitness professionals in a locked room to formulate an exercise program for one particular person, you would end up with five different exercise programs. Yet, the reality is, they could all make good sense. That's because there are many ways to get physically fit. The road to becoming fit may incorporate many different types of exercise equipment or none at all. The <u>frequency</u> of exercise (*how many times per week*), the <u>duration</u> of exercise (*length of time performing the exercise*) and the <u>intensity</u> of exercise (*the ease or difficulty at which you perform the exercis*e) may vary widely, yet the results may be the same - that the person participating in the program becomes physically fit.

The exercise program, which I am about to present, has been used by me to train people of varying levels of ability over the past twenty-five years. While I have been involved in training football players and Olympic athletes, the majority of my training experience has been in the clinical setting, evaluating and designing exercise programs for weight management and at risk patients. In the mid-1970's, I directed the Laboratory of Applied Physiology at the Cardiac Rehabilitation Center in Miami. Patients stayed with us for 28 days, during which time we taught them how to exercise, eat right and reduce stress. The program was so successful, statistically we returned 80% of our patients to gainful employment. This program was one of the first comprehensive lifestyle modification or <u>wellness</u> programs in the country.

Unfortunately, at that time, most insurance companies and the Social Security Administration were of the opinion that people suffering from heart problems could not be rehabilitated. Back then, third party reimbursements for cardiac rehabilitation services were very sporadic, leaving the bulk of these bills to be paid for by the patient. This made the cost of cardiac rehabilitation too high for the majority of people who desperately needed these services. In a sense, insurance companies and the government were more willing to cure a broken leg - than a broken heart. Today, many of these same programs are completely reimbursable. It took quite some time for them to figure out that <u>it's a great deal more cost-effective to cure a damaged heart than pay for long-term hospitalization or disability</u>.

When I first started out in this field, my original orientation was towards designing cardiovascular exercise programs to promote good health. I was a firm believer that cardiovascular (*aerobic*) exercises were the key to good health and possibly to increasing longevity. Years later, I came to realize that neuromuscular (*strength*) training was equally important. I now know that a combination of cardiovascular and neuromuscular exercises coupled with stretching is the most effective format to gain and maintain physical fitness.

When beginning an exercise program, I want you to forget the slogan, *No Pain - No Gain*. I want you to remember that, if you feel any moderate or sharp pain while exercising - <u>slow down and stop</u>. We're not teenagers or trained athletes anymore. Our bodies need time to adjust as we begin an exercise program. There are no shortcuts, just pitfalls. The single biggest pitfall is trying to get fit fast. It took time to get out of shape and it will take time to become physically fit. Remember, instead of the slogan *No Pain - No Gain*, you might substitute a more sensible slogan:

'When in Pain – Refrain'

What you wear while exercising is important. I'm not telling you to run out to the Mall to buy a new wardrobe. As a general guideline, wear loose comfortable clothing made from a breathable fabric. Never wear heavy, tight clothing or clothing made from a plastic or vinyl material that doesn't allow sweat to evaporate off your body. It's natural to sweat and this sweat serves an important purpose while you exercise. It helps to keep your body cool. Take a moment to lick the back of your hand - now blow on it. Feels cool, right? As sweat evaporates off the surface of your skin, it cools the blood near the surface. The blood that was cooled continues to circulate throughout your body, cooling the internal organs. This evaporative cooling process is known as <u>convection</u> and is an important way your body keeps from over-heating while exercising.

So now you know the basics of how to approach a program of regular exercise. You have to:

- Do it for the right reasons
- Start slowly
- Let your body gradually adjust to the exercises
- Dress appropriately
- Drink plenty of water

The time has come for you to take those first steps towards …

Getting Back to <u>BASICS</u>.

Develop a Healthy Heart

In the mid-1970's, at the Cardiac Rehabilitation Center in Miami, members of our professional staff developed a speakers bureau. Several evenings each month we would travel around to condominiums and senior citizen residences lecturing on the topic; A Total Approach for a Healthy Heart. Our team included a cardiologist, registered dietician, psychologist and exercise physiologist. We spoke about how members of the audience needed to make controllable risk factor lifestyle modifications in order to stay healthy. We told them that they had a very simple choice; An ounce of prevention or a pound of cure.

Surprisingly, when we first began these free lectures, only 10 or 15 people would attend. This low turnout continued for quite a while until a Miami businessman, who happened to be a patient of ours, made an interesting observation. Having attended one of our condominium presentations he said, *'If I were you, I would charge people to attend your lectures.'* The other staff members and I were shocked at his recommendation. We naturally figured that if only 10 or 15 people showed up for a free lecture, no one would attend lectures if they had to pay. Reluctantly, we agreed to try his suggestion and we soon found out that he was right. Our audiences now contained over 100 people willing to pay and were interested in what we had to say. Some time later, when I asked him why this was so - he said, *'People always believe they get what they pay for. If it costs nothing - it can't be very good.'*

Now that I think of it, I am fairly certain that most people are of the opinion; you get what you pay for. The thought process of the human mind tends to put a perceived value on things. While a free lecture may have no perceived value, somehow, a paid lecture may raise the credibility of the speakers, because we may perceive it as being worth more. I know, it's a little confusing, and I may be l rambling a bit, but this leads me to an interesting observation concerning how we may perceive the benefits derived from an exercise program.

Whether a person continues to participate in an exercise program, or quits, may depend upon how quickly our brain perceives changes in our appearance. It's possible that when we go to the gym for the first time, our subconscious brain may be telling us, *'Now that you started exercising and taking such good care of yourself, you can expect to see some real changes in your appearance because everyone knows - you get what you pay for.'* I wouldn't be surprised if some people expect to see a dramatic change in their appearance as they leave the gym after their first workout. Sadly, in life, many of us have been conditioned to expect immediate gratification and if it's not there - we quit.

But that's not the way it is. Physiologically, the changes, that take place when you begin an exercise program, begin at the cellular level. You won't notice them at first because all the good stuff that's going on would require an electron microscope to observe. If you give it a little time, you will probably begin to notice subtle changes at first. You know, those pants feel a little looser, or you're able to walk up the stairs without becoming breathless. In order for a program of exercise to bring about changes that you can see in the mirror, you have to give it at least 4-6 weeks.

It's been proven that cardiovascular (*aerobic*) exercises increase the strength of contraction of your heart muscle and the efficiency of transporting blood and oxygen to every cell in the human body. Cardiovascular exercises include brisk walking, jogging, stair climbing, aerobic exercise classes, cycling, upper body ergometry, swimming, cross-country skiing, among others. To achieve significant benefits, these exercises must be performed for a varying amount of time, with your heart rate climbing to a specified target heart rate range. While performing cardiovascular exercise, it's a good idea to measure your heart rate before, during and after exercising, to ensure that you're working at the proper level of intensity without over-doing it. If you're not sure how to measure your heart rate read on.

How To Measure Your Heart Rate

First you'll need a watch or clock with a second hand. You are going to measure how many times your heartbeats each minute. Begin by placing the palm of your right hand face up. Take the fleshy tips of the three middle fingers of your left hand and place them on your right wrist approximately 1 inch below your right wrist, on the thumb side. If you've done this correctly, you will probably feel some slight pulsations. Count the number of pulsations you feel for a period of 15 seconds. Multiply that number by 4 to get your heart rate. If you felt 20 pulsations in 15 second your heart rate would be 80 beats per minute. Before you begin to exercise, check your heart rate to make sure that it is not too low or too high. It should be somewhere between 60 and 80 beats per minute. If you've been sedentary for a long period of time and your heart rate prior to exercise is below 60 or above 80, you should check with your doctor before you begin your exercise program.

Your heart should beat in a rhythmic pattern. If you find that your pulse is irregular before exercising check with your doctor. If your pulse is irregular at any time while exercising, slow down, stop and again check with your doctor. If however, you just don't feel right while exercising, you take your pulse, and find that it is irregular you should <u>seek medical attention immediately</u>.

Calculate your Target Heart Rate Range

I mentioned earlier that in order to achieve optimal benefits while performing cardiovascular exercises, your heart rate must climb to a specified target heart rate range. This range is based on your age. The older you get, the lower your target range. To calculate your individual target range, subtract your age from the number 220, then multiply the result by a percentage of you maximal predicted heart rate. Usually this percentage will range between 55% and 85% (*of your maximal predicted heart rate*) and is based on your current level of physical condition. This percentage will determine the intensity of your cardiovascular workout. If you've been physically inactive - use 55% to 65% to determine your range. As you get in better shape, you might increase the percentage to 70% or 75%.

> **Formula to Determine Target Heart Rate Range** (at 70% Level)
> Target Heart Rate = (220-Age) x 70%
> *If you're 53 years old - To exercise at the 70% level*
> (220-53) x .70 = 116.9 bpm *(round to 117)*
> Your THR Range would be 107-117 bpm

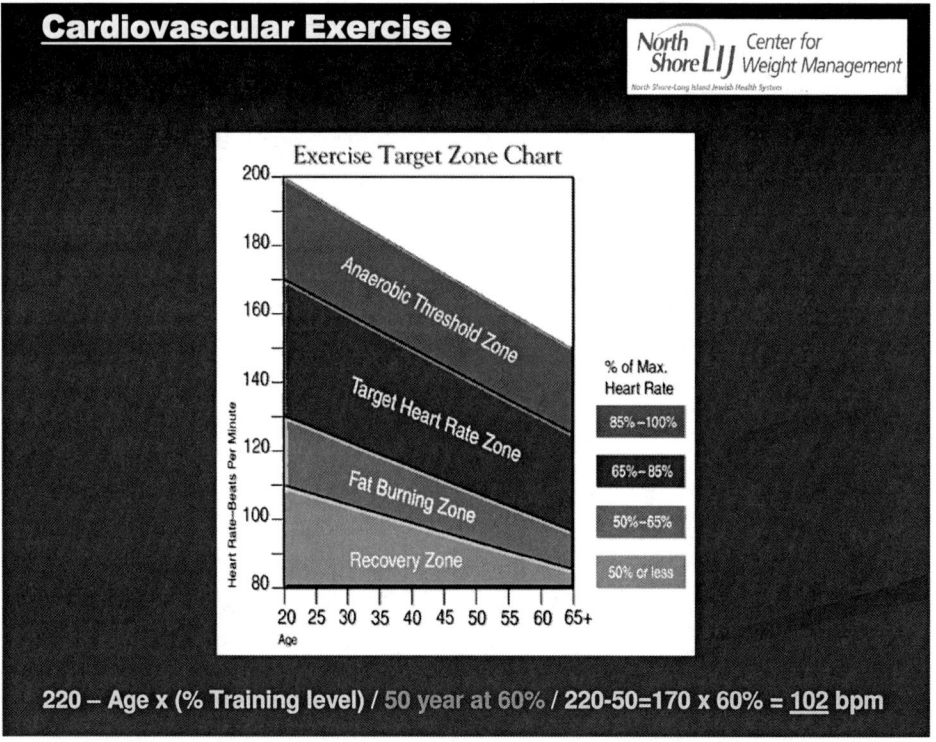

Page 46

Rated Perceived Exertion

Some of you out there in <u>babyboomer land</u> may find it difficult to take your pulse while exercise. I admit it's not easy to do. However, there is a way to judge the intensity or difficulty of your exercise session without having to measure your heart rate. This method is called <u>Rated Perceived Exertion</u> or (RPE). While you are exercising you have to stay in touch with your feelings. When you begin to exercise, you are doing so at an easier intensity. You're not breathing as hard and your pulse is relatively low. As you increase your exercise intensity you will breathe more rapidly and your heart rate will climb. When you reach your target zone your respiration and heart rate will be faster and you should be able to note this difference in the level of your exertion. Using the Rated Perceived Exertion scale you rate the level of difficulty of each stage of your exercise session on a 1 to 10 scale, with (1) being the lowest level of intensity and (10) the highest. Some people use other numbers, but I find (1 -10) the easiest for people to remember. As you exercise more frequently, you should become better at judging the intensity of your workouts (1-10) based on your perceived feelings. While this rating system is a valuable tool, I am more comfortable when people also learn how to measure their pulse rate and pulse rhythm.

Some Words Of Caution

Many of us are currently taking medications for high blood pressure or irregular heart beats. Many of these medications are <u>beta-blockers,</u> which decrease your heart rate and increase the strength of contraction of your heart muscle. These and some other prescribed medications may prevent your heart rate from reaching your target range, no matter how hard you try. It's very dangerous to attempt to raise your heart rate to your target range when you are taking medication, which lowers your heart rate.

If you were currently taking any drugs for high blood pressure or some other heart medication, check with your doctor to find out what heart rate level would be a good starting point when you begin to exercise. If you have someone supervising your exercise program, tell your trainer if you're taking a beta-blocker, or any other heart medication. If they look at you funny as if to say, *'Why are you sharing this with me?'*

<u>It's time to find another trainer.</u>

I mentioned earlier that while performing cardiovascular exercises you should strive to raise your heart rate to your predetermined target range in order to achieve optimal benefits. <u>Not everyone will be able to reach this range</u>. When you begin your exercise session, you must start out slowly and gradually increase the intensity of the exercise to allow your body enough time to adjust to the physiologic changes, which take place. Your heart rate will increase, your breathing will become deeper and faster and your arteries will vasodilate (*widen*) to allow more blood and oxygen to move to the working muscles efficiently. This is a normal response to exercise.

The initial time interval of aerobic exercise is called the warm-up. I generally recommend that people warm-up for at least 5 minutes. During the warm-up period your heart rate should gradually rise as you increase the intensity of exercise. For example, if your cardiovascular exercise were brisk walking, you would gradually increase the speed of walking to increase your heart rate during the warm-up period.

Once your heart rate reaches your target heart rate range you are in the training zone. If you've been inactive, I would suggest that you stay in the training zone for only 5 or 10 minutes, then begin to slow down. As you become more physically fit you would gradually extend the time in the training zone. It's not uncommon for a person who has been exercising regularly to spend 30 or more minutes in their target zone. As you begin to slow down, you are cooling down. The cool-down allows your body to adjust back to its pre-exercise state and should last 5-10 minutes.

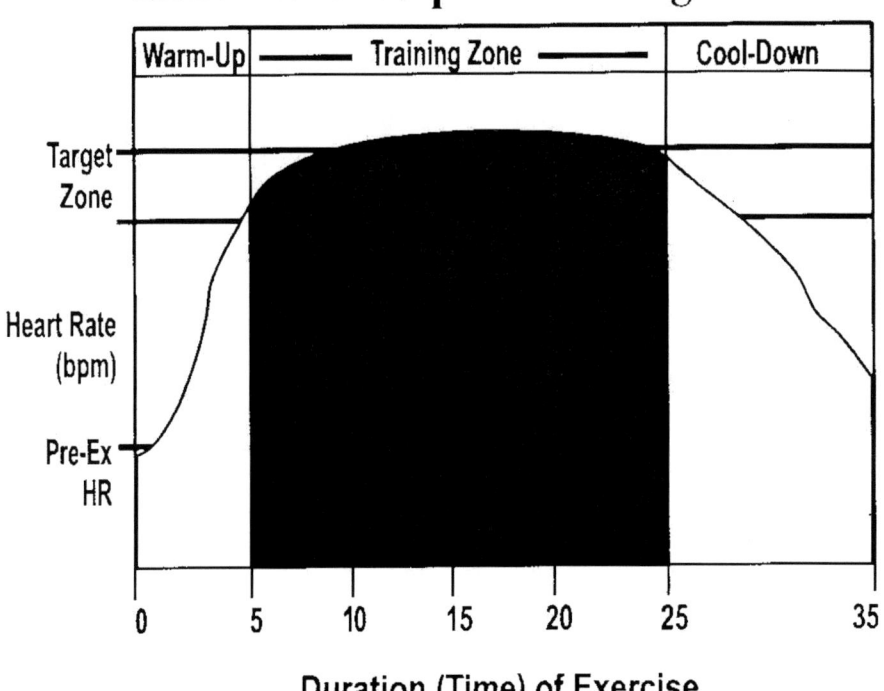

The graph on the preceding page highlights the normal heart rate response during cardiovascular exercise. As you begin to exercise your heart rate should be relatively low. As you warm-up your heart rate gradually increases. If you exercise at a high enough intensity your heart rate will probably reach your training zone. Not everyone will be able to reach this zone. If you're taking prescribed medication, consult with your doctor to determine your appropriate heart rate training zone. When you complete your time in the training zone, you reduce the intensity of exercise as you cool-down.

Let's Begin to Walk

It's been projected that over 20 million Americans would consider themselves regular walkers. <u>The American Heart Association recommends walking 30 - 60 minutes, four to six times each week or 30 minutes daily</u>. When starting a walking program, I suggest that you:

- Stretch before and after walking

- Start slowly and gradually increase your speed

- Keep your stride natural

- Wear sneakers or appropriate footwear

- Let your hands swing naturally at your sides

- Set a comfortable pace and don't compete with other walkers

- Don't stop abruptly, gradually slow down when done

From a historical perspective, you've probably heard that the earliest humans walked on all fours. Then one day, an enlightened ancestor decided to make a change and here we are upright, prone to low back problems but a whole lot better looking. In making the change from <u>quadra-pedalism</u> (*walking on all fours*) to <u>bi-pedalism</u> (*walking upright*) our body had to make some unique anatomical adjustments. The 206 bones of our skeletal system and our muscles had to adapt to our upright posture. It's sort of interesting to note that our bodies went through these dramatic postural changes, all because some primitive ancestor decided we wouldn't look good walking on all fours once we started wearing - <u>designer clothes</u>.

Well, the time has come to dust off your treadmill and remove the clothing from the handrails. If you're just starting out, try 5-10 minutes of brisk walking at a comfortably slow speed without elevation. The important thing to remember is that you can always raise the speed. In the beginning, don't worry about trying to raise your heart rate to your target heart rate level. You have to give your body time to adjust. If you try to go too fast in the beginning, you will significantly increase the risk of hurting yourself. After a few workouts, if you still feel good, you may gradually increase your treadmill time and speed. After awhile, as you become more physically fit, you may add some elevation (*1% or 2% grade*) to increase the intensity of your workout. If you're walking outdoors you may try walking up some small hills to increase the intensity of your walk.

10,000 Steps Can Save Your Life

I consider brisk walking to be one of the best cardiovascular exercises. While owning a treadmill is a big plus, if you don't have one there's always the local high school track or indoor walking at the mall. If you're just starting out, track your daily step count using a pedometer. Track and record your step count for one week, then calculate your average daily step count. The following week try to increase your daily count by 250 – 500 steps. You can download a free *Step Log* at the Get Fit For Life website – www.MyTrueAge.com. In addition to all the healthful benefits of walking, according to many research studies, '*increasing your activity level will significantly decrease your risk of premature death.*'

<u>Now that's a benefit I can live with.</u>

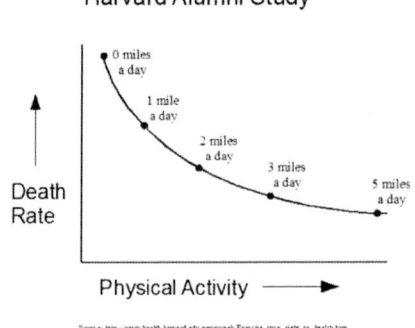

Sensible Guidelines For Resistance Training

In the late-1980's I owned a large health club in Fort Lee, New Jersey. It was a luxury club, which catered to everyone, not just body builders. One day while I was working out at the club, I observed one of the few serious body builders lifting 40-pound dumbbell weights in each hand. He was a rather large individual doing the biceps curl exercise with 40-pound dumbbell weights, while I was doing the same exercise with 10-pound dumbbells. You've probably guessed that I'm the type of person who likes to joke around with people. Sometimes they like it, occasionally they don't. But seeing this body builder lifting 40-pound dumbbell weights, I just couldn't help myself. At some point, I jokingly said, '*you know, my mother does that exercise with the same amount of weight.*' He smiled and without missing a beat replied, '*no wonder, she's been raising a dumbbell all her life.*' In one fell swoop my joke backfired, and I became my mother's - dumbbell son. After that, the two of us broke down laughing.

I'm glad we were both laughing. In hindsight, I realize that it was not such a good idea to joke around with a body builder holding two 40-pound dumbbell weights, when you're a featherweight baby boomer.

While some fitness professionals might disagree with me, I believe, '*whether you are working out at the gym or exercising at home, you don't need expensive exercise machines to get fit. Properly used dumbbell weights can give you a better workout than most exercise machines.*' I base this statement on several facts I have come to accept over the years:

- Weight machines are manufactured for people of varying size, but have inherent design limitations. If you're very short or very tall you may not fit the machine properly. In addition, something as simple as not setting the seat adjustment properly can alter the biomechanics of the movement and can result in injury.

- When you lift dumbbell weights there is no stabilization of the weight. Theoretically, as you lift a dumbbell it could drift off in any direction. Each hand must move the weight in the desired direction and stabilize it at the same time. In order to accomplish this more muscles must be called into action. By involving more muscles during each dumbbell exercise you get a better workout.

- Most weight machines require you to push or pull a single weight bar with both hands. If you're right handed, you may use more effort with your dominant right hand to lift the weight. In doing so, muscles on the right side of your body get a better workout. When lifting dumbbell weights, each hand moves independently, allowing the muscles on both sides of your body to get an equal amount of work.

- If you're working out at your gym during peak hours, <u>you may have to wait to use exercise machines</u>. If the gyms crowded and you can't get on your favorite exercise machine, don't use that as a convenient excuse to leave. Instead, 'Don't be a dumbbell – *<u>use the dumbbells</u>*.'

- Lastly, <u>weight machines are usually too expensive to purchase for home use</u>. You can buy dumbbell weights very inexpensively and you don't need a lot of room to store them. If you already have a treadmill, several pairs of dumbbell weights are all you need to help you get fit and stay fit.

<u>CAUTION</u>: If you're just beginning a resistance-training program and you have been physically inactive – <u>check with your doctor</u> – before you start.

The importance of resistance training as an integral part of your exercise program, stems from strong medical evidence, which suggests that - <u>participation in strength conditioning programs may help to reduce your risk of Osteoporosis</u>. As we age our bone density decreases, which makes bones more susceptible to breaks. Even simple slips and falls can result in broken bones for people who suffer from Osteoporosis. It's widely believed that a properly formulated resistance-training program may slow this decline.

Another benefit derived from your participation in a resistance-training program may be that it reduces joint and muscle pain. These pains may be attributed to a prior injury or an arthritic condition. Nevertheless, over the years, many times I have heard program participants say, '*I can't believe that my shoulder, hip or knee no longer hurts.*' As muscles become stronger, they play an increasingly important role in stabilizing joints. It may be this added stability, which provides the relief.

I know as soon as I mention the words resistance-training *(strength-training, weight training)* some men may say, '*I don't want to become Mr. Universe, why lift weights?*' - or women may say, '*I don't want to get muscles like a man.*' In both cases you needn't worry. The program I am about to present uses light dumbbell weights to increase muscular strength and endurance, enabling you to perform your daily activities with less effort.

If you're just starting a resistance-training program, listed on the following pages are general guidelines, which will help to reduce your risk of injury.

Resistance-Training Guidelines

- Begin with a very low weight
- Do not exercise the same muscles every day
- Lift weights with slow, controlled movement
- When you lift a weight do not hold your breath
- Stay well hydrated
- Do not ignore symptoms of intolerance

Lets take a few moments to examine these guidelines

Begin With A Very Light Weight

This may sound like a very logical guideline, almost not worth mentioning. Unfortunately, many first-time exercisers injure themselves by attempting to lift weights that are too heavy. In the beginning, it's always better to err on the side of too little, than too much. If you're really out-of-shape, you should start with a very light amount of weight. I would recommend no more than 3 or 5 pounds. While you might be thinking to yourself that you're capable of lifting much heavier weights, I don't advise it. Your muscles, tendons and connective tissue need time to adjust to resistance training. If you start with a weight that's too heavy, you might injure yourself and you're back to square one and not exercising.

During your first resistance training session, try to perform each of the exercises 12 times (reps). If you feel all right the next day, wait one additional day and try it again doing 15 repetitions. During subsequent sessions increase the repetitions gradually, only if you feel good between sessions. When you are able to do 20 repetitions for several sessions, you may be ready for the next higher weight. When you increase to the next weight level, decrease back to 12 repetitions and gradually increase the repetitions over a period of time. <u>I'm a firm believer that as we get older we should limit the amount of weight we lift and increase the number of repetitions.</u>

As you train, you will find some exercises more difficult than others. You should not expect to increase the amount of weight and reps for all of your exercises at the same pace. If you're working out at a gym, don't look at other people and try to copy what they're doing. An exercise that's appropriate for one person may be dangerous for you. Remember: It took time to get out-of-shape and it will take time to get back into shape. You cannot rush the process.

Do Not Exercise The Same Muscles Every day

Your body needs rest as much as it needs to exercise. At the end of your weight training session the energy level of the muscles you worked-out are at their lowest level. Over the next 24 to 48 hours the energy level is replenished. Biochemically, the breakdown process is known as <u>catabolism</u>, while the replenishment, or restorative process is called <u>anabolism</u>. For this reason, you should only workout a particular muscle on an alternate day basis. For example, if you did the biceps curl on Monday, wait until Wednesday to perform the same exercise. If you don't allow muscles sufficient time to recuperate, you increase your risk of injury. Your body needs rest, as much as it needs exercise. The problem is, some of us are really good at the rest part - and terrible when it comes to doing the exercise.

Lift Weights With Slow, Controlled Movements

If you've been to a gym recently, chances are that you saw someone throwing a weight up in a pumping action. While that training method may be fine for athletes or body builders, it's not good for casual exercisers or baby boomers. In a weight-training program, <u>it's not how much weight you lift</u> - <u>it's how you lift the weight</u>. Technique is the most important consideration. Good technique will maximize your benefits and reduce the likelihood of injury. Bad technique will do the opposite.

Weight training should always be done with slow, controlled movements. If you throw the weight to get it up, the initial muscular spurt develops momentum, which propels the weight, taking much of the effort off the muscle. If you were training for a particular sport that required explosive movement, this might be all right, but if you were working out to get back in shape, this would be a dangerous way to train.

Anatomically, muscles are made up of tiny muscle fibers. With proper training, the diameter of these muscle fibers increase in size and the muscle gets bigger. To get the best results, you want all the muscle fibers of a particular muscle to '*fire*' as you exercise the muscle through its full range-of-motion. In order to accomplish this, every muscle fiber must be called into action when lifting a weight. If you throw a weight to lift it this doesn't happen, reducing the effectiveness of your training.

When You Lift A Weight Do Not Hold Your Breath

This guideline is so important, that if you don't do it right you could end up in the hospital. Whenever you lift a weight or any heavy object <u>DO NOT HOLD YOUR BREATH</u>. Sounds pretty serious. That's because it is. If you hold your breath and physically exert at the same time, you perform what's known as a <u>valsalva maneuver</u>. This may significantly increase your risk of elevated blood pressure, irregular heartbeats, stroke or heart attack.

One way to prevent holding your breath while resistance training is to breathe out when you lift the weight. Some people say you should, <u>blow the weight away</u>. I ask patients to count the number of repetitions as they lift weights. This forces them to breathe out as they exert. You cannot breathe in and talk at the same time. As you say the number while lifting the weight, you reduce the likelihood of performing a valsalva maneuver.

Stay Well Hydrated

Just as you need to replenish fluids when doing cardiovascular exercises, you need to do the same while weight training. Some health clubs and most home gyms are not well ventilated, which will substantially increase your fluid loss. If you don't consume a sufficient amount of fluids while exercising, you may become dizzy or disoriented. When training outdoors, do not exercise in extreme heat and humidity. Whenever you exercise, to prevent a heat related disorder, stay well hydrated.

Do Not Ignore Symptoms Of Intolerance

Your body has a way of letting you know when you are doing too much. <u>Unfortunately, many of us become deaf when we should be listening to what our bodies are telling us</u>. I hear stories from patients who had heart attacks, telling me that they knew they were doing too much, yet in spite of the fact that they did not feel well, they still didn't pay attention to the early warning signs. Whenever you perform any physical activity - if you feel dizzy, disoriented or pain in any part of your body not generally associated with the activity - **<u>slow down and stop!</u>** If you ignore the symptoms of intolerance you run the risk of heart attack, stroke, injury or worse. When you begin an exercise program you have to use good common sense <u>and listen to your body</u>.

Some Final Words Of Caution

While it may not always be possible, <u>I strongly advise everyone beginning an exercise program to workout with a partner</u>. Exercising with a friend or significant other may help to motivate you, and keep you on track. In the unlikely event that you're not feeling well, your exercise partner is someone who can assist you.

Illustrated Resistance-Training Program

Appendix A (*beginning on page 103*) illustrates some of the dumbbell exercises that I have found work well for people just beginning a resistance-training program. While these exercises have worked well for many, you and your doctor are the best judge of whether or not these exercises are appropriate for you.

Keep Well Hydrated – Drink Water

When it comes to selecting the best natural fluid for a healthy body, water is the hands-down winner, without exception. Did you know that your body is almost three-fourths water? You may not realize it, but maintaining proper water balance in the human body is essential for maintaining good health. It's so important that you probably wouldn't last one week in the absence of water. Yet, so many of us don't drink enough water. Instead, we walk around in a state of near dehydration, usually constipated, generally irritable and most probably, less healthy than we could be.

Water is an integral part of all bodily functions. It is essential that we continually replenish the supply of this life-giving fluid. In a sense, water is nature's gift to humanity.

There's nothing that will quench your thirst better than water, yet many people don't drink it. They prefer sugar-laden, carbonated drinks or alcoholic beverages to satisfy their taste buds. Many of these drink substitutes provide empty calories and artificial flavors just to make them palatable. What most people don't realize is that, a significant amount of the excess sugar we consume each day comes from liquids we drink. You could save yourself a lot of money and unnecessary calories by switching to plain, old-fashioned, thirst quenching, and life-giving water.

Almost 75% of our human body is comprised of water. Is it any wonder that approximately 72% of our entire planet is made up of water? The same fluid that gives life to our planet gives us life. Without water this planet would be a rock, nothing more. Without water we would die, nothing less. Yet, without enough water, we may live, but our bodies would not, and could not, perform at an optimal level of efficiency.

Water is such an important component of our lives that even slight variations in the amount we consume and lose can lead to serious, if not fatal consequences. Most of us are under the erroneous belief that our body's thirst mechanisms will alert us before we become dehydrated. Unfortunately, this is not always the case. Under extreme circumstances it's possible to lose great amounts of fluid and become severely dehydrated quickly and without warning.

Almost every football season we hear a horror story about a high school, college or professional athlete who died of heat stroke because they exercised under extreme conditions and did not consume enough replacement fluids. I am certain that emergency room physicians could tell us countless stories about non-athletes who made the same mistake. In almost every case these were preventable.

As I mentioned earlier, the evaporation of sweat off our skin and a thermal regulatory process called convection, is the major way our body cools itself while we exercise. As we become dehydrated, our ability to sweat decreases and our body temperature rises. <u>Even mild dehydration may lead to impairment of mental judgment and coordination</u>. If the condition does not improve, changes in the delicate balance of electrolytes caused by the loss of sodium and chloride ions would eventually lead to heat exhaustion. The loss of sodium chloride (*salt*) is one reason why it may be a good idea to drink a sports drink like *Gatorade* if you must be physically active under extreme conditions. Salt tablets are not recommended because they are too concentrated and draw water away from the circulatory system where it's needed, and into the stomach to dilute them. While heat exhaustion is not a life threatening condition, if left untreated it can lead to heat stroke, which is. Perhaps the most important thing to remember is, <u>if you must perform physical activity under extreme conditions of high heat and humidity - drink because it's necessary</u> - <u>not because you're thirsty</u>.

If these are not good enough reasons to have you increase the amount of water you drink each day, consider the following:

Drinking Water can help you Lose Weight

> Drinking water is a good way to suppress those nasty *I'm hungry* messages your appetite center frequently sends you. Sometimes when you become dehydrated, your brain becomes confused and sends you an *I'm hungry* message, instead of an <u>*I'm thirsty*</u> message. If you can't tell the difference, you'll tend to eat, instead of drink. Your body will absorb some water from the food you eat, but if it's not enough, you'll keep getting mixed signals to eat, when your body is really saying - <u>drink water</u>.

Stretching May Prevent Injuries

It's common knowledge that being in good physical shape will reduce your risk of injury when you participate in any type of physical activity or roll around on the floor with your grandchildren. While most sports authorities agree that stretching is an important component of any physical conditioning program, they also agree that it's often the most neglected.

Good flexibility permits the joints to go through a greater range-of-motion, and may reduce the likelihood of injury to muscles, joints and connective tissue. While most of us know that stretching may be valuable before and after exercise, the reality is, most people don't stretch - and if they do - they do it wrong.

All babies are born flexible, however, only some of us maintain good flexibility throughout our lives. As we age, our bodies adjust to the level of physical activity to which we have become accustomed. If we've been physically inactive, our bodies conform to that level. If we stay in good shape, we're less likely to suffer those inconvenient muscle strains, pulls or tears. In order to maintain good flexibility you have to stay active and stretch.

If you don't use it ... you'll lose it!

Before you stretch, I recommend some light cardiovascular exercise for about five minutes. This will allow your muscles to warm up and be better prepared for stretching. As you start to stretch, you should stretch to the point where you feel some tightness (*initial stage*). If the tightness melts away, increase the stretch just a little. This little extra, (*developmental stage*) helps to increase flexibility.

Never bounce as you stretch. This is a common mistake we probably learned in high school. The act of bouncing over-stretches the muscles and connective tissue. If you've ever played with a new rubber band and continually pulled on it, you would notice that it could never return to its original shape. If you pulled too hard, it would break. If you bounce while stretching you could do the same thing.

Many fitness professionals question whether or not stretching prevents injuries. While there is little hard evidence that it does, many athletes believe it helps. I believe that cold muscles are more likely to tear than warm ones and that the warm-up prior to stretching, and the stretching itself, may help to prevent injuries.

There are many books and articles written which describe in great detail how to increase your flexibility through proper stretching. One of the best is <u>Stretching</u> by Bob Anderson. Another great way to improve flexibility would be to enroll in a stretching or yoga class.

'Risk Change - Overcome Fear ... And Win'
Unknown

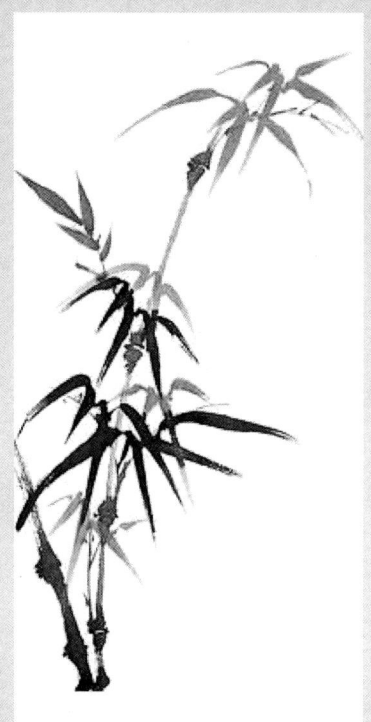

Part 5

Manage Stress To Stay Healthy

You Can't Separate The Mind From The Body

Manage Stress Or Suffer Distress

You Have To Keep Your Sense Of Humor

A snapshot of
What the current economy is doing to us

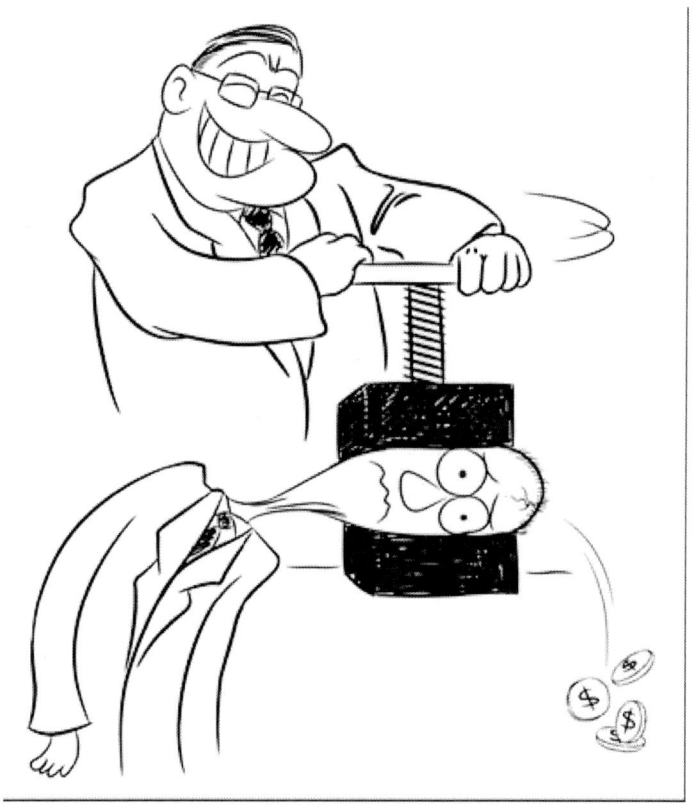

Trust me ... this will relieve the stress.

The Mind/Body Connection

You can't separate the mind from the body. The French tried with the guillotine, but the results were disastrous. Many physicians report that a significant number of their patients who come to them thinking that they are sick, have no organic sickness at all, rather, they suffer from some mental distress that has triggered a physical symptom. Have you ever suffered palpitations during a stressful event? At one time or another, most of us have experienced some physical symptom in response to excessive mental distress.

What's even more interesting is the fact that those of us who think we are sick generally get sick, just as those of us who think we are old appear to be old. The mind is a powerful tool in gaining and maintaining good health. If you constantly think of yourself as sick, you can create that condition in your body. It's also true that if you continually see yourself as healthy, you can greatly improve your general health. If you don't think this is true then answer this question, why do placebos work? How could a sugar pill cure a particular health problem? The fact is the pill may have done nothing, cured nothing. It might have been your belief that the pill could cure, that created the circumstances for your own body to cure itself. In essence, it might be a case of mind over matter.

Ninety years ago, Arnold Lorand, M.D. an eminent physician and researcher of his day published a book entitled, <u>Old Age Deferred</u> in which he wrote, '*It is my intention to show, that premature old looks can often be caused by faulty habits; such as not drinking a sufficient amount of water or having a diet consisting mainly of meat, fats, milk, butter and sweets. This is the surest road to obesity. To stay healthy preference must be given to a diet with a small amount of meat and larger amounts of green vegetables and fruits.*' Dr. Lorand continued, '*Less injurious than sport is walking. It is desirable to walk as much as possible, and never use a street car or a carriage unless pressed for time; by this means health may be greatly improved.*'

It's interesting to note that living according to the Basic Laws of Health is not new information. Dr. Lorand and many others before him stressed the importance of living within the Laws of Health for hundreds of years. They knew the importance of eating right, exercising, drinking enough water and obeying the Basic Laws of Health. What was true then is equally true now. However, today it is much more difficult to live life according to the Basic Laws of Health. Why is it more difficult? Because in our civilized culture - the same technological conveniences that have reduced our need and desire to stay physically active, have also reduced the nutritional value of most of the foods we eat, poisoned much of the water we drink and significantly polluted the air we breathe.

Recently, while having a discussion with a cardiologist friend of mine, the topic turned to the great advancements in life extension that society has seen this century. We discussed how the average life span of someone living one hundred years ago was probably close to forty-five years. How a person living just fifty years ago could expect to live until age sixty and that today, the average life span is in the mid-seventies. The cardiologist argued that with continued research and the development of new drugs, treatments and anti-aging hormone supplements, we could expect the life span to increase to one hundred years or more. While I agreed with some of his argument, I disagreed with him giving full credit for the substantial increase in life expectancy based purely on scientific discoveries, vitamins and hormone replacement therapy. My argument was that one hundred years ago, people lived less stressful lives than they do today. They generally ate foods closer to nature, not containing food additives with excessive salt and sugar. They were more physically active and depending upon where they lived, they may have breathed cleaner air. So why then was their life expectancy much lower?

Back then, people died from typhus, cholera and other diseases we have essentially eradicated in America today. Many people died young because they did not understand the importance of good hygiene and proper sanitation. The reason we live longer today is in part due to the fact that people no longer die from many of the diseases that plagued our ancestors. Imagine what life might have been one hundred years ago if people did not have to suffer and die from those diseases. Chances are that the average lifespan would have been much greater than forty-five. In fact, if we were able to apply some of the amazing medical advancements of today 100 years ago - I speculate that their life span might have been longer than ours is today.

Within the last decade there has been a controversy brewing in the medical community concerning the effectiveness of hormone replacement therapy. Many doctors swear by them in the belief that, as we age, various hormone levels decline in our bodies. They believe that this hormonal decline accelerates the aging process, while hormone replacement therapy decelerates or reverses the aging process. I believe that the verdict is still out concerning the effectiveness of hormone replacement therapy. It's nice to believe that the fountain of youth may be found in a pill or injection; however, the field of Anti-Aging Medicine is too new to place all of your eggs in one basket.

While there may be controversy concerning the use of hormone replacement therapy, there is no controversy concerning eating healthy foods, sleeping soundly, exercising regularly, drinking plenty of water, thinking positively, managing your stress and not smoking or using excessive alcohol or abusing drugs. These healthful lifestyle modifications are time-tested winners in helping to turn back your biological clock. Down the road, it's possible that replacement hormones may help you to stay healthy and live a longer life. In the meantime, you must focus your attention away from what might be in the future, to the realization that you still have to make healthy lifestyle choices right now.

This century has seen marvelous almost miraculous advances in the science of medicine. Who could have envisioned organ transplants just fifty years ago? While these miracles of medicine have saved countless lives, there is a dark side - that the public has come to expect that science will eventually cure all of humanities health problems. Today, many of us look for the quick and easy cure for most illnesses. Often these quick fixes compound the problem making the original problem more difficult to cure.

It's been said that we live in a *pill-popping* society. Today, many of us believe, *'if I get this - I should take that.'* So much so that, at the first sneeze, many of us rush to a doctor to get a shot or a prescription. While some medications are helpful, and some essential, the fact remains; all too frequently we over-medicate ourselves. This tendency to over-medicate can result in serious medical complications caused by drug interactions. While one might be quick to blame the doctor for this problem, in reality, many patients literally force their doctors to prescribe these medicines. Frequently patients seeking a quick cure for minor illnesses, demand a pill or injection from their doctor, and if not satisfied with their doctor's response, find another doctor willing to comply.

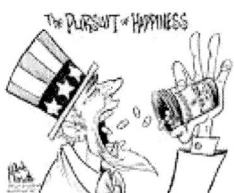

It's possible that our pill-popping cultural philosophy is partly the result of our widespread misconception concerning the effectiveness of certain medications. Somehow we have developed the erroneous belief that all drugs and medicines cure disease. The reality is, <u>many of the over-the-counter medicines we take, and some prescribed medications, mask symptoms but do not cure illness</u>. Often, when a doctor prescribes a medication for a particular illness, the relief of symptoms experienced by the patient is mistaken for a cure. In most cases, it's your body's own curative powers that restores your health and sets the wrong right. Perhaps Oliver Wendell Holmes, M.D. (*yes, he was a Medical Doctor*) put it best, <u>yet a little extreme</u>, when he wrote, *'If most of the medicines in the world were thrown into the sea, it would be bad for the fish - and good for humanity.'*

Manage Stress or Suffer Distress

You just got home from an exhausting day at work. It's raining outside and you're still upset from something your boss said earlier in the day. You can count the days until your retirement. You close your umbrella and hang up your coat, glad to be back on your home turf. You sit in your comfortable chair to take a moment to relax, then suddenly life changes. The phone rings. It's your daughter, complaining that the babysitter was delayed and there's no one to watch your grandchildren when she goes to graduate school. Could you help? By the way, the youngest was complaining that he wasn't feeling well. You rise to grab your coat and notice that the dog left a deposit on the carpet. You get to your car and it doesn't start. You begin to feel the stress level rise as you get more and more worked up.

We've all had days like these. You know, those days we would like to forget. Yet, at times like these, we get a true picture of how we handle the pressures of life. At one time or another we all have had bad days. '*How we deal with the emotions of this type of day will determine whether we manage stress or suffer distress.*'

There's no avoiding the fact that stress is a part of our complex world. It comes with the territory and we just have to deal with it. When we deal with it effectively, we generally stay healthy. When we let it take control of our lives, we usually suffer distress and become unhealthy.

Thousands of years ago, early humans had to survive in a primitive world. When someone left their cave to hunt, it was at great risk to them. Often, the hunter became the hunted. Their instinct for *fight* or *flight* helped them to decide, whether it was a good idea to pursue a fight with a particularly fierce animal or run away to fight again another day. It's apparent that stress played an important role in human existence from the dawn of humankind, helping our earliest ancestors evaluate and react to dangerous situations.

In modern times, you might be driving along a highway. It's a beautiful, sunny afternoon and you seemingly don't have a care in the world. You're totally relaxed as you cruise along at 60 miles per hour. Then, out of nowhere, a tractor-trailer cuts you off, like you weren't there. You jam on your brakes to avoid a collision and hope that no one is tailgating you. For a brief moment, your heart stops, you can't breathe, as you feel the adrenaline rush sweep over your body. Just as suddenly as it appears, it's gone, the danger passes and you slowly return to normal. What you experienced might have been the same feelings that early humans experienced during a dangerous encounter with a fierce animal. While primitive people probably had no words to describe those feelings, today one might call it an episode of acute stress.

Acute stress is an almost instantaneous reaction to a very stressful situation. The effects are quick and at a high intensity. When the danger passes, the body begins to calm down, usually with no long-term health effects. However, in extreme cases, it's not uncommon for people to suffer heart attacks or strokes in response to these very stressful moments.

On the other hand, chronic stress is a more insidious type of stress that will damage your health. Chronic stress is characterized by long-term release of stress hormones that can cause high blood pressure, heart attack, stroke, memory problems or other related health disorders. It is this type of stress, which we must learn to deal with in order to stay healthy. The long-term effect of chronic stress - is distress.

Chronic stress is caused by many factors including, work problems, financial worries, relationship challenges, child-rearing difficulties - the list goes on. In today's uncertain world, it's almost impossible not to be affected by bouts of chronic stress. So what can you do to avoid it? Simply stated, there is no way to avoid it. You have to learn to deal with it. You have to learn different coping skills, which will allow you to keep a lid on mental stress, so that you don't blow your top, causing physical distress.

Did you know that hotheaded people are much more prone to heart attack and stroke than their calm counterparts? It seems that the very act of getting angry and losing our temper dramatically increases our risk. We should have known, since for a very long time, we knew that Type A (*highly excitable, driven*) people are more likely to suffer heart attacks and strokes then Type B (*relaxed*) people. The next time you start to lose you temper because someone stole your parking space or jumped ahead of you on line say to yourself, '*Is it worth it to get so upset?*' The answer is, no!

 I tell my Type A friends and patients, you need to learn to vacillate within a finer emotional range. By that I mean, when good things happen, you can be happy, but don't go way overboard. On the other hand, when bad things happen, you cannot become overly depressed. Happiness and sadness are a part of our lives. You must learn to control your emotions and not vacillate between emotional peaks and valleys. Life should not be an emotional roller coaster.

On a somewhat lighter note, as we get older we tend to forget things. Most of us appropriately call these times, senior moments. We all have them, some of us more frequently than others. I recently read a joke on the Internet I'd like to share with you.

> It seems an elderly couple went to the doctor because they were concerned about their memory. The doctor examined them and told them that their problem was not serious, however the solution would be to write everything down. That evening the couple was watching television and the husband stood up and started to leave the room. His wife asked, *'where are you going?'* He replied, *'to get some chocolate ice cream.'* The wife said, *'I'd like some too - <u>write it down</u>.'* The husband hearing this said, *'Honey ... its only chocolate ice cream - I can remember that.'* As he began to walk away his wife added, *'put some whipped cream on mine - <u>write it down</u>.'* The husband immediately replied, *'chocolate ice cream and whipped cream I can remember that.'* Again, he started to walk away as his wife called out, *'don't forget a cherry on top - <u>write it down</u>.'* At that point the husband became a little testy as he replied, *'chocolate ice cream, whipped cream and a cherry on top - I can remember that.'* Without hesitation off he went to the kitchen. Thirty minutes later he came back to the room with two plates of bacon and eggs. The wife looked at her husband in utter amazement and said, **'<u>You Forgot The Toast</u>.'**

Hopefully your memory is not quite that bad. However, if you find that life is a little more overwhelming for you now than it used to be, you might consider trying what I do when I absolutely have to remember something.

<u>WRITE IT DOWN</u> - *that's no joke!*

Believe it or not, lists are good. You might consider placing items on the list in some order of priority. If you absolutely have to do something, and can't afford to forget it, put it at the top of the list. You don't have to do everything on the list. Break the list down into do-able amounts so that you don't get over-stressed. Things that can wait until tomorrow, or the next day - can wait until tomorrow or the next day.

To avoid chronic stress you have to exercise regularly, eat right, stop smoking and get plenty of sleep. In addition, you have to take some time for yourself to unwind. You might read an enjoyable book, paint, take a walk in the park, listen to your favorite music, do something for you. Don't think about doing it - <u>just do it</u>.

I once asked a college class what was the difference between the words <u>living</u> and <u>existing</u> and saw a lot of blank faces. Many thought the words meant the same thing. The fact is, when we get up, have breakfast, go to work, come home, eat dinner, watch some television, then go to bed - we <u>exist</u>. When we break the routine and do something different, something we like to do, something that makes us feel alive - we <u>live</u>. In order to keep stress from turning into distress you have to take some time for yourself and - <u>live a little</u>.

You're having a bad day. You feel the stress mounting as your body tightens up. Your head is pounding, the headache is incredible and it's only 9 a.m. in the morning. At times like these you have to take some immediate action to reduce the stress, before it overpowers you.

If you're feeling stressed right now, you might consider trying a relaxation technique I use when I get a bit overwhelmed. First, I find a nice comfortable chair, preferably in a room where I can dim the lights. I close my eyes and try to imagine a beach I visited several years ago. I let the vision of the white sand against the bright blue ocean waters flood my mind with feelings of peace and serenity. Palm trees sway in the breeze as I imagine the wind gently caressing my face. As I visualize this special place, I take a deep breath and hold it for 2 seconds. With my lips almost closed, I gently allow the breath to slowly exit my mouth as I think to myself the word, 'c-a-l-m.' Sometimes, when I'm too busy and cannot get away from my desk, I stare at some object on the adjacent wall and practice this same breathing technique without closing my eyes.

In today's economy it's not easy to deal with the stressors of daily life. However, there are some strategies you can use to help you control stress. Listed below are some good techniques to keep stress from becoming distress.

Techniques To Prevent DISTRESS

1. Try To RELAX Whenever possible take mini-breaks. Sit in that comfortable chair and try the deep breathing exercise I mentioned. Another way to help you relax and get a better handle on stressful situations would be to learn the technique of diaphragmatic breathing available at the Cleveland Clinic website listed below:
  [http://www.cchs.net/health/health-info/docs/2400/2409.asp?index=9445]

2. Practice Acceptance Many people become upset over things they don't accept in themselves and others. While you might be able to change things about yourself, you can't change someone else's feelings or beliefs. You have to learn to accept those things, which are outside your power to change, or at least act responsibility when dealing with them.

3. Avoid Dangerous Situations You have to rationalize the impact of stressful situations on your health. Is a particular situation dangerous? If the answer is _yes_ then remove yourself from it immediately.

4. Organize Yourself Design a reasonable schedule of daily activities that includes some time for you. Make a daily To Do List. Try to be as productive and efficient as possible.

5. Exercise I can't say it enough - exercise reduces stress. We live in an age of conveniences that has severely limited our need and desire to be physically active. Most of us sit behind a desk or at a computer terminal to earn a living. Stress builds up because of our inactive lives and we need an outlet to prevent it from becoming distress. Exercise is the answer.

6. Smell The Roses Many of us are part of the rat race and seldom get a chance to smell the roses. If you're the type that's always checking the time, try to take things a little slower. Recognize that you can only do so much in a given period of time. You have to learn to <u>PACE yourself</u> - <u>don't RACE yourself</u>.

7. Be Calm - Not Combative Every life situation should not be approached from a combative or competitive position. Whenever possible try to tone it down. Don't raise your voice when it's not needed. Stay in control at all times and approach life from a calm perspective.

8. **Special Time** Whenever you get a chance, schedule some time for yourself. Relax in the tub, listen to some good music, take a walk, read a book, chat with family members and friends. These special times are important to help you keep the proper balance in your life.

9. **Get Back To BASICS** Making healthy lifestyle modifications will help you to reduce stress in your life. By conquering fears and breaking some bad habits, you raise your self-image and greatly improve your self-esteem. This will go along way towards helping you to meet the stressful demands of our increasingly complex world.

As I mentioned earlier, we all have to deal with stress. We need a certain amount of stress in our daily lives to function normally. As a positive influence, stress can compel us to take action and give us that creative spark. As a negative influence it can lead to feelings of anger, rejection and depression. Long-term chronic stress will lead to serious health problems.

It's interesting to note that there is no single optimal level of stress for all people. Each of us handles stress in our own way. One person may love to handle stressful challenges and arbitrate disputes on the job, while another is more comfortable in a relaxed, stable work environment. For some of us, sitting at a desk shuffling papers is relaxing, while others have a compelling need to be out and around. In order to handle stress properly, we need to find that optimal level of stress, which will motivate us to a higher level of personal accomplishment, without overwhelming us.

During my years at the Cardiac Rehabilitation Center in Miami, I had the opportunity to talk to many patients who made the mistake of taking themselves too seriously. Their entire life, to that point, was geared towards making money, becoming successful. Not surprisingly, even while many of these same people were lying in a hospital intensive care unit after having a heart attack, some were more concerned about their work than their health. I often wondered why a person so close to death would place work above all else.

Only now am I beginning to understand that for many of us our work is a mirror image of who we are. We may be failures in many areas of our lives, but if we are successful at work, somehow we are successful at life.

Unfortunately, for many people, their work is their life. Over the years they have honed business skills, gained appreciation, respect and responsibility only to have it taken away when they retire. For some, this is a bitter pill to swallow. While many retirees maintain active lifestyles following their retirement, many do not. If your life before retirement focuses around work, to the exclusion of other interests and hobbies, I suggest that you think very carefully before you retire. You must begin to develop other interests to keep your mind active and your spirits up. If your self-worth is tied to the workplace, maybe you need to rethink your retirement plans.

Stress or Distress - <u>that is the question</u>. We all have to deal with it. No one can escape it. What you have to realize is that the things that stress you, stress all of us. You're not unique in your feelings. You're part of the family of humanity who had to deal with the stressors of life from the beginning of humankind. Maybe in some way it's comforting to know that you're not alone. We all have to deal with the same stressors in life. There are effective strategies to keep stress from becoming distress. As you learn to deal effectively with stress, you take another positive step towards …

Getting Back to <u>BASICS</u>.

<u>Health Tip</u>

> Years ago my mother cooked with a pressure cooker. It sat on top of the stove and had a cylindrical shaped pressure valve cap on top. When it was being used, the cap would make a rattling noise as it released built up steam. Over the years, I've come to realize that, in our complex world, life is often a pressure cooker. At times, we all need to lighten up a bit and release some steam in order to stay balanced. While a vacation to some exotic location may not always be possible, a trip to the zoo, a get-together with friends, or a quiet walk in the park, will help you to release steam enabling you to relax and enjoy life.

Keep Your Sense Of Humor

> A cardiovascular surgeon calls a plumber to fix a leaky facet. When the plumber was finished he presents the doctor with a bill for $150.00.

<u>Doctor</u>: *One hundred and fifty dollars to fix a leaky facet in fifteen minutes? I'm a cardiovascular surgeon – and I don't make that kind of money.*

<u>Plumber</u>: *Well – when I was a cardiovascular surgeon – neither did I.*

I hope you're laughing, or at the very least chuckling, at the above joke. If not, it's time to look at the humorous side of life. Up until this point, I've talked about how you have to make healthy decisions in order to stay healthy. Now, I'm telling you that, in order to stay healthy, you need to fine-tune your sense of humor.

Throughout history, oppressed people have often poked fun at their plight in life, using humor as a means to exercise some degree of control over the chaotic conditions they were forced to endure. In doing so, they may have helped their bodies to maintain a physiologic and mental balance. The fact is – <u>humor may be the way our body insulates itself from the mental wear and tear of daily existence</u>.

I'm sure we can all name some people who don't appear to have a sense of humor. I suspect that many of these people are not only unhappy - they may also be unhealthy. It's possible that life has dealt them a physical or emotion blow they are unable to recover from. Their feelings of hopelessness and despair may make them unwilling to change, triggering a downward spiral in their health. If this is the way you view yourself right now, then the time has come for you to face up to the fact that you're not alone. Many other people have felt what you feel. Some are able to get past those feelings of loss, while others remain anchored to the depths of despair. The question is, how are some people able to free themselves and rise above those destructive feelings? Part of the solution may be through: <u>humor</u>.

<u>Humor is powerful medicine that doesn't cost one penny</u>. It's good for the mind, good for the soul, and good for the body - and it has no adverse side effects. I mentioned earlier that the mind plays a powerful role in how we perceive the state of our health. I said, if a person thinks they are healthy, they generally are healthy, and if a person thinks they are sick, they can cause themselves to get sick. The fact is humor is a powerful ingredient in helping one to maintain a positive mental outlook.

Humor has been used in medicine throughout recorded history. One of the earliest mentions of the health benefits of humor is in the book of Proverbs in the Bible. As early as the 13th century, some surgeons used humor as a distraction during surgery. Today, there's even an emerging therapeutic field known as humor therapy to help people heal more quickly. While available scientific evidence does not support the use of humor as an effective treatment for any disease, research has shown health benefits from laughter ranging from strengthening the immune system to reducing food cravings to increasing one's pain tolerance.

Humor therapy uses the power of smiles and laughter to assist healing. Often called therapeutic humor, it helps find ways to make people smile and laugh. An example of humor therapy would be clowns performing in the children's ward of a hospital cheering up sick children. Some hospitals even have humor carts that provide funny materials for patients of all ages.

Scientists in a field called psychoneuroimmunology have been researching the relation between the mind/body - and its' ability to promote healing. Their research indicates that laughter appears to change brain chemistry and may boost the immune system. It may be that humor allows a person to feel more in control of a situation thereby making it seem more manageable. Laughter allows people to release fears, anger, and stress, all of which can harm the body over time. Humor improves the quality of life and is good medicine.

The Benefits of Laughter

- Hormonal: Laughter reduces stress hormones like cortisol, epinephrine (adrenalin) and dopamine.

- Emotional: Laughter provides both a physical and emotional release.

- Physical: Laughter exercises abdominal muscles, the diaphragm, upper arms and shoulders and may benefit the heart.

- Stress: Laughter is a de-stressor that changes your focus away from negative emotions and anger.

- Social: Laughter is contagious and connects people. It provides an opportunity for positive social interaction and helps to moderate stressful situations.

So how does a person develop or fine-tune their sense of humor? That's a simple question with a simple answer - <u>by learning how to tell a joke</u>. I can't tell you how many times I've heard people say to me, *'I love jokes but I just can't tell them,'* or *'I just can't remember the jokes people tell me.'* The truth is, the people who tell jokes are no different than the people who love to hear them, with one exception. The people who tell jokes took a little time to practice them and commit them to memory.

I remember years ago, when I directed the cardiac exercise program at the Bayside Medical Center, I was often called upon to train foreign doctors in the nuances of cardiac and stroke rehabilitation. They were all extremely bright doctors who learned quickly, but had one slight problem. In a clinical setting, they often had difficulty making patients feel at ease. Occasionally, it may have been due to a language problem, other times it was a cultural difference. However, most of these doctors felt that they had to maintain a stern demeanor, and that it was inappropriate to tell a joke to a patient. It's quite possible that some American born doctors feel the same way. However, I've always felt more comfortable with a doctor who could smile and tell a joke at an appropriate moment, than the serious stoic.

To complete the training of these foreign doctors, I felt it important to teach them the value of having a good sense of humor. I would give them a joke, which I wrote out for them, then told them to practice it in front of a mirror at home. The next day I would allow them to tell the joke to patients in the exercise room, and I would give them pointers on their delivery. Most often, the delivery was funnier than the actual joke. The patients would howl with laughter and the foreign doctors and I would laugh as well. Invariably, they would tell me that, this one lesson helped to make their patients feel more comfortable in the antiseptic clinical setting.

So, what's the proper way to tell a joke? There is no one correct way. Everyone develops his or her own style. Just remember, people like to laugh. They enjoy having someone make them smile, often in the face of hardship or adversity. In learning to tell a joke, you improve your health and make others feel good - as you take another crucial step towards …

Getting Back to <u>Basics</u>.

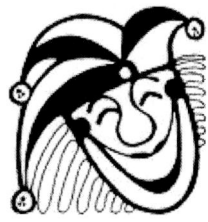

How To Tell A Joke

1. You have to memorize it. There's nothing worse than beginning a joke and forgetting the punch line. I call that '*jokus-interruptus*.'

2. Now try to tell it out loud in the privacy of your home in front of a mirror.

3. You have to pace your delivery by speaking very slowly and rhythmically. Don't race through the joke or people will not understand what you're saying.

4. Speak clearly and occasionally change your volume. Don't speak in a monotone or everyone will be asleep when you're about to deliver the punch line. Instead of laughing, they'll be snoring. This is not the response you're after.

5. Maintain eye contact and smile often. If there are several people listening, change the direction of your eye contact so that everyone feels that they are getting some of your attention.

6. Try to stay at ease. The whole idea of telling the joke is to make the other person feel comfortable. You cannot do that if you look uncomfortable. Relax, and '*go with the flow*.'

7. When you're done, hopefully everyone is laughing with you. However, if they're laughing '*at you*' don't feel bad. Remember, the whole idea of telling the joke was to break the tension. Any laugh is better than no laugh at all.

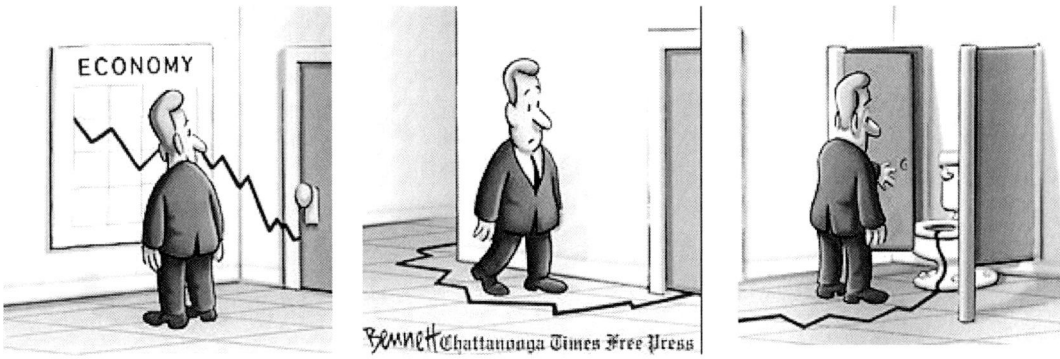

Remember ... You have to keep your sense of humor

Here's a short one you can practice in front of the mirror

> An eighty-three year old lady just completed her annual physical examination when her doctor said, Sadie, you're in great shape for a woman your age, but tell me ... do you still have intercourse?
>
> Just a minute, I'll have to ask my husband, was her response. As the puzzled doctor scratched the back of his head, Sadie headed for the waiting room to see her husband.
>
> Morris, do we still have intercourse? She bellowed so that all could hear. And Morris replied: I told you once; I told you a thousand times ...
>
> We have BLUE CROSS.

Remember: As with anything else in life.

Practice, Practice, Practice

My father was a milkman and had a wonderful sense of humor. He always had a joke to tell and was an expert at his <u>delivery</u> of both <u>milk</u> and <u>jokes</u>. He taught me everything I know. As I was growing up, my father and I had some standard jokes that we really enjoyed. Some of them were rather lengthy and took too much time to tell. To solve that problem, my father and I numbered certain jokes. A <u>#3</u> might be the one about the unfaithful husband, while a <u>#6</u> might relate the story of the forgetful old man. We got so good at numbering our jokes that we no longer had to tell the joke. At the appropriate time, I might yell <u>#3</u> and the two of us would start laughing uncontrollably. I remember on one occasion, while we were talking about some event of the day, I really felt that a <u>#17</u> joke would be perfect for the occasion. I patiently waited until just the right moment and yelled out <u>#17</u> as loud as I could to which my father replied:

<u>You told it wrong!</u>

*'You must begin to think of yourself...
As becoming the person you want to be.'*
David Viscott

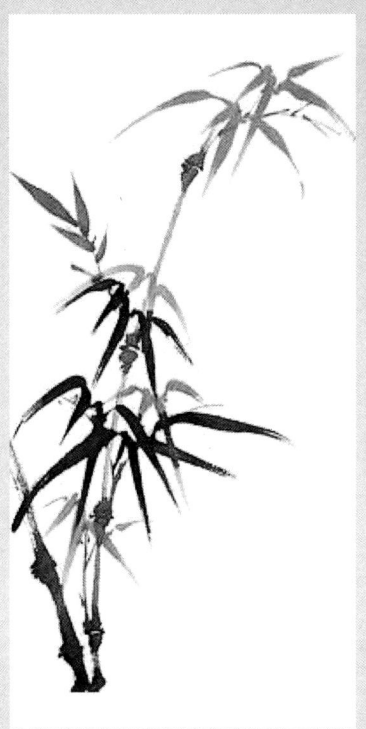

Part 6

The Importance Of A Good Nights Sleep

Sleep Soundly

10-Tips For Better Sleep

Sleep Problems In Children

The Economy Of Sleep

A study of sleep patterns by the National Sleep Foundation, a non-profit organization that promotes a better understanding of sleep, found that up to one-third of Americans are losing sleep because of the current economic instability in the United States. The study also suggests that poor sleep patterns have a strong correlation with unhealthy lifestyles, and that those of us who get enough sleep, are twice as likely to exercise, eat healthy foods and maintain good health.

Personal finances, unemployment and health care costs are near the top of the list of what keeps people awake. However, concerns about the economy and your financial situation should not cause you to sacrifice sleep. Sleep is essential for productivity and alertness and is a vital sign of one's overall health. Lack of sleep has a profound impact on your ability to function impairing judgment, focus and reaction time.

With the exception of sleep apnea and narcolepsy, most sleep issues are caused by stress and bad habits. As you continue to read this book and make healthy lifestyle adjustments, you may sleep better as you take another important step towards …

Getting Back To **BASICS**

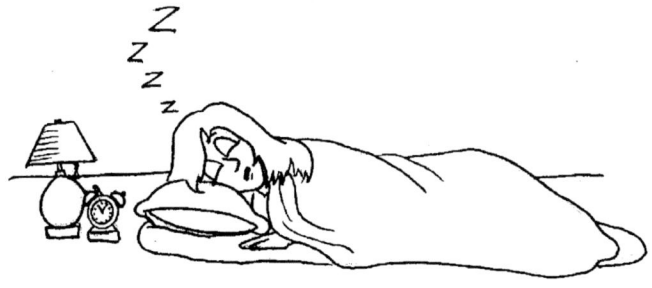

Sleep Soundly

Sleep deprivation is a common disorder among all groups of Americans. While some of us, burn the candle at both ends; others just find it difficult to get to sleep. Either way, you may wake up in the morning feeling just as tired as when you went to bed. You spend your day in a sluggish stupor, never fully waking up, feeling as if there was something radically wrong with your body. The fact is there is something wrong. If you go to bed at a reasonable hour, sleep erratically and wake up tired, I suggest that you speak with your doctor. Occasionally, this may be due to a more serious medical problem or a side effect of some medication.

While we generally need less sleep, as we get older, the average adult requires between six and seven hours of uninterrupted sleep each night. The body uses this time to rebuild itself and replenish the energy, which had been used up the preceding day. By denying yourself necessary sleep, for whatever reason, in essence you are robbing yourself of good health.

Some of us fool ourselves by saying, I only need fours hours a night. Even if this was true, the fact remains that you would not be allowing your body enough time to recover from the day before. Instead of giving your body the proper sleep time necessary to replenish itself and get stronger, you continuously deplete your physical energy, which will cause you to get weaker. While you might get away with this for a short time, over an extended period of time, you would probably pay the price. Unfortunately, the price is usually a bed in some hospital's intensive care unit.

There are many reasons why people have difficulty getting to sleep and staying asleep. Sleeplessness may be caused by stress, foods you eat or drink prior to bedtime, smoking or exercising too late at night. Sometimes, after a particularly stressful day at work or at home with the children, we keep replaying the events of the day, over and over again, making it difficult for us to relax. In a sense, we've become so wired we can't unwind. It's well documented that sleep patterns change, as we get older. Usually it takes longer to get to sleep, our sleep is not as deep and we may wake up several times during the night.

It's believed that 50 to 70 million Americans chronically suffer from a disorder of sleep and wakefulness, hindering daily functioning and adversely affecting their health and longevity. The long-term effects of sleep deprivation have been associated with a wide range of health problems including; increased risk of hypertension, diabetes, obesity, depression, heart attack, and stroke.

Lack of sleep can be expensive: Each year, billions of dollars are spent on medical costs associated with doctor visits, hospital services, prescriptions, and over-the-counter medications as a direct result of sleep disorders. The National Commission on Sleep Disorders estimates that sleep deprivation costs $150 billion a year in higher stress and reduced workplace productivity.

Consequences of Sleep Deprivation

- **Decreased Performance and Alertness**: Sleep deprivation causes a significant decrease in performance and alertness. It's been suggested that reducing sleep by as little as one and a half hours a night could result in a reduction of daytime alertness by as much as 32%.

- **Memory and Cognitive Impairment**: Decreased alertness and excessive daytime sleepiness will impair memory and cognitive ability - hindering your ability to think and process information correctly.

- **Relationship Stress**: Sleep disorders may be responsible for relationship problems due to excessive moodiness and irritiability causing marital strife.

- **Occupational Injury**: It's been shown that sleep deprivation contributes to a much greater risk of occupational injury.

- **Automobile Injury**: The National Highway Traffic Safety Administration (NHTSA) estimates that drowsy driving is responsible for at least 100,000 automobile accidents, 71,000 injuries, and 1,550 automobile fatalities each year. It's believed that almost 20 percent of all serious car crash injuries are associated with driver sleepiness.

According to Lawrence Epstein, president of the American Academy of Sleep Medicine, *'we have in our society this idea that you can get by without sleep and not suffer any consequences... we're finding out that's just not true.'* While many aspects of sleep remain a mystery, including exactly why we sleep, it appears that not sleeping enough runs counter to the body's internal clock, throwing a host of basic physiologic functions out of sync. Unfortunately, we have nothing in our biology that allows us to adapt to this behavior.

Physiologic studies suggest that sleep deprivation may put the body into a state of high alert, increasing the production of stress hormones driving up blood pressure, a major risk factor for heart attacks and strokes. Moreover, people who are sleep deficient have elevated levels of substances in the blood which indicate a heightened state of inflammation in the body, a major risk factor for heart disease, stroke, cancer and diabetes.

If you have a really good mattress, but you're still having problems getting to sleep, listed below are 10 suggestions, which may help:

10-Tips For Better Sleep

1. Develop a bedtime routine that helps you to relax both mentally and physically.

2. Stick to calm, non-stressful activities prior to bedtime. Read a relaxing book or listen to calm music.

3. Avoid caffeinated beverages, nicotine, and alcohol and limit your intake of fluids, prior to bedtime.

4. Check with your doctor to find out if sleeplessness is a side effect of any medication you are currently taking.

5. Avoid napping during the day.

6. Avoid action movies or suspenseful books just prior to bedtime.

7. Try taking a warm bath or shower to calm you down prior to bedtime.

8. Do not exercise several hours before bedtime.

9. Keep a pad next to your bed to write down things that are on your mind.

10. Keep your bedroom quiet, dark and at a comfortable temperature.

Sleep Problems In Children

If your child has difficulty concentrating in school or has become more irritable than usual, it may be caused by sleep deprivation. Often, lack of sleep is the cause behind unusual mood swings or diminished performance in school academics or athletics.

According to James Kemp, MD, medical co-director of the Pediatric Sleep Laboratory and Sleep Medicine at St. Louis Children's Hospital. *'While adults may suffer from daytime sleepiness due to inadequate sleep, children tend to become hyperactive when they are overtired. If your child is acting differently and appears to be highly distractible, try getting him to bed an hour earlier for a week. If this doesn't work, talk with your child's pediatrician about other possible solutions.'*

Develop A Bedtime Routine

For young children, sleep requirements can be met, in part, through naps. Naps are important for toddlers and should be part of their daily routine. Small children are constantly processing newly acquired information, and naps allow their brains to rest and reset, providing a positive benefit for learning and development.

When it comes to establishing a bedtime routine, children need structure to help them maintain a regular schedule. To help make bedtime an unstressed event, parents should not let children have caffeinated drinks less than six hours before going to bed, and should turn off the television, video game or computer one hour prior to bedtime.

According to Sharon Bathon, RN, sleep nurse coordinator at St. Louis Children's Hospital, *'To help your child become accustomed to a routine, you must set rules before bedtime and stick to them. If you go to your child every time he or she cries, they will continue to do so. Assure your child that you are there for them, but let them know bedtime is not negotiable. In time, they will stop fighting you and understand it's just a part of their day.'*

If your older child resists going to bed at night, remember this; it's your parental responsibility to put your child to bed, but it's your child's responsibility to get to sleep. If you put your child to bed at a reasonable time, but they don't fall asleep, it may be because - some children need less sleep than others.

*'Though no one can go back and make a brand new start ...
Anyone can start from now and make a brand new ending.'*
Carl Bard

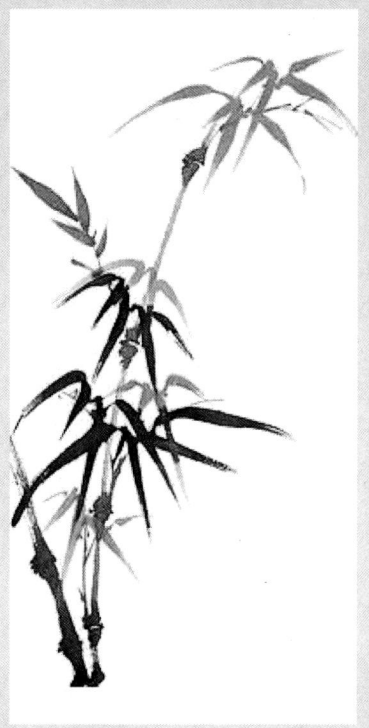

Part 7

The Unlikely Piece Of The Wellness Puzzle

Manage Your Money To Stay Healthy

The Impact Of Today's Economy On Your Health

Recreate Your Destiny By Putting The Pieces Together

Gaining and maintaining good health is as simple as putting the pieces of the wellness puzzle together - each piece representing a risk factor that must be controlled. In today's world, all of us must take a serious look at our own puzzle and decide which pieces are connected and which are not. As we join the pieces of the wellness puzzle together we improve our health taking another significant step towards ...

Getting Back to <u>BASICS</u>.

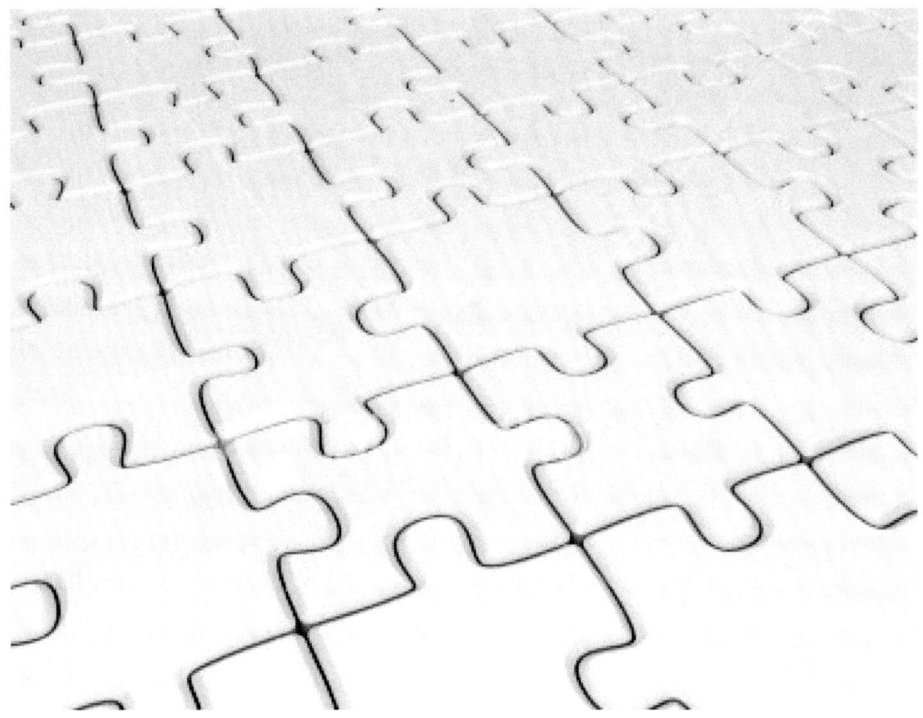

The Wellness Puzzle

Manage Your Money To Stay Healthy

You've never heard of the Wellness Puzzle? Don't feel bad, most people haven't. I started using the word wellness back in 1975 at the Cardiac Rehabilitation Center in Miami. Back then, the word was so new that very few people understood its meaning. Today, the word *wellness* is well known and has become infused in our health and *wellness* cultural vocabulary.

Years ago, when I lectured for the Cardiac Rehabilitation Center, I would begin by telling the audience they had choices in life. Healthy lifestyle choices would exert a positive influence on the quality of their lives, while poor health choices would result in a decline in health. In a sense, their options were, an ounce of prevention ... or a pound of cure.

As I continued my lecture, I explained that we all have risk factors which impact the state of our health and may predispose us for certain medical conditions. Some risk factors are beyond our control (i.e. age, hereditary) and are often called uncontrollable risk factors. Others, controllable risk factors, are within our power to change.

This book is all about Controllable Risk Factors

> We can do something about the way we eat. We can stop smoking. We can increase our level of physical activity. We can learn how to deal with excessive stress. We can drink plenty of water. We can learn how to control the habitual use of drugs and alcohol. We can modify poor or risky health habits and substantially influence the quality of our lives. We can do all of these things, if we're properly directed and properly motivated.

As I ended my lectures, I spoke about the Wellness Puzzle. Think for a moment of the word *wellness*. Now think of that word fragmented into small pieces like a jigsaw puzzle, each piece of the puzzle representing one controllable risk factor. If all the pieces of the puzzle were connected, by living a healthful lifestyle, the word wellness would emerge and we would experience optimal health. If, however, the pieces of the puzzle remained fragmented by a disjointed, unhealthy lifestyle, we would experience poor health. I reminded them back then, as I remind you now that, within each of us is the power to exercise some degree of control over the destiny of our health. If we can somehow learn to put the pieces of the Wellness Puzzle together, we can improve our quality of our lives – and perhaps live longer.

You might be thinking, why did he name this chapter, *The Unlikely Piece of the Wellness Puzzle*. That's because most health practitioners rarely, if ever, consider the topic I am about to present as having anything to do with a discussion of controllable risk factors. Maybe they're right, but I think not.

It's that time of the month again that fills many of us with a sense of uneasiness. You know, that time most of us dread almost as much as going to the dentist for root canal work. It's time to get out the checkbook and pay the bills. There, I've said it, that awful B word.

I know you're thinking to yourself, where is he going with this. Has he totally lost his mind? Don't worry, I'm still somewhat sane, and if you permit me a moment, I may be able to bring it all together so that it makes some sense.

Whenever I lectured on the topic *An Ounce of Prevention ... or A Pound of Cure*, I would mention how controllable risk factors are lifestyle issues that influence our health. I would stress the fact that, since they are classified as controllable, we can change them. If we're properly motivated, we can learn how to eat right, exercise, quit smoking, etc. So where does money management fit into the equation? I call it, *The Unlikely Piece of the Wellness Puzzle*. It not only fits into the equation, we should consider it a *big-time* risk factor that must be properly managed in order to stay healthy.

Have you ever-lost sleep wondering where you're going to get the money to pay the mortgage? car payment? tuition? I know, I can almost hear some of you saying, cut it out, you're making my blood pressure go up. That's just the point. The mere mention of that B word, and our body begins to tighten up and squirm. I think you'll agree that money management is a critically important risk factor that we must learn to deal with effectively.

Like clockwork each month, most of us sit down to the often-unpleasant task of trying to meet our expenses and pay the bills. Sometimes the bill paying session is easy, the money is there. Sometimes it's not and we must find inventive ways to make or stall payments. I remember someone once saying to me, at the end of the month, after paying the bills - if you still had $1.00 left over - that's HAPPINESS. If you were short $1.00 - that's SADNESS.

If, at the end of the month, after paying those nasty bills, we still come up short, what options do we have? As far as I can tell, basically two, the first being to find ways to increase your income, without resorting to bank robbery. The second would be to learn how to manage money better. While some of us may have options for increasing our monthly income, others may just need to learn how to manage what we already have.

I can almost hear some of you saying, *'what's with this guy. I'm 56 years old, with three children and six grandchildren, and he's going to tell me how to budget my money?'* No, I'm not about to tell you how to manage your money if you have your finances under control. However, it may come as no surprise when I tell you that most people don't live within budget. In fact, most families don't even have a budget. In some cases, that's because they have found a natural balance to make ends meet, without having to put things down on paper. Their income always exceeds their expenses and every month they have a few dollars left over that goes into savings. Unfortunately, for a great many families of all ages, this is not the case. For them, bill-paying day is a traumatic event and money problems are a constant burden, which impact on their health and happiness. If you find yourself in the latter circumstance some or all of the time, pay particularly close attention to the following section.

First of all, I want to remind you that I'm not a financial planner, stock broker, accountant, banker or Walmart cashier. I'm only a clinical exercise physiologist who is not the best person to give advice on money matters. So why am I doing it? Simply, <u>because no discussion of health risk factors would be complete without exploring the relationship between money and health</u>.

Let's begin by trying to get a handle on your <u>FINANCIAL FITNESS</u>. In order to do this, you'll need a large piece of paper, a pencil and calculator.

First - You are going to list all of your monthly expenses divided into three separate categories:

Category 1. <u>FIXED EXPENSES</u>
These are monthly expenses that cannot be delayed or changed. They may include: mortgage, rent, loans, insurance, etc.

Category 2. <u>PERIODIC EXPENSES</u>
These are monthly expenses that you may be able to reduce. These may include: credit cards, telephone, utilities, etc.

Category 3. <u>DISCRETIONARY EXPENSES</u>
These are purely optional expenses and should be the first to go if you're in a financial pinch.

Your monthly expense list might look something like this

FIXED EXPENSES
Mortgage $_____
Car lease $_____
Home Insurance $_____
Tuition loan $_____
Real Estate Taxes $_____
_____ $_____
_____ $_____

PERIODIC EXPENSES
Credit Card(s) $_____
Telephone(s) $_____
Utilities $_____
Food - at home $_____
Food - eating out $_____
Medical $_____
Clothing $_____
Car Expenses - gas/maintenance/repair $_____
Transportation - bus, cab, etc. $_____
Personal Grooming $_____
_____ $_____
_____ $_____

DISCRETIONARY EXPENSES
Entertainment $_____
Snack foods (*cookies, candies, etc*) $_____
Frequent manicures and pedicures $_____
Expensive vacation $_____
New luxury car $_____
Stereo system (*best money can buy*) $_____
_____ $_____
_____ $_____

While you might categorize a particular item as discretionary, someone else may itemize it as periodic. If you're having a problem at this stage, it only confirms the fact that you really need to see a qualified financial advisor.

It's time to take a realistic look at your monthly income. Don't look at the gross amount on your check; that's not what you take home. Use the net pay amount you make on a monthly basis. If you and your wife work, use the combined net income monthly. If you have a second job or other income sources, add these net amounts to determine your total monthly net worth. Now, let's calculate your FINANCIAL FITNESS.

Calculate your FINANCIAL FITNESS

(1) Enter your   TOTAL MONTHLY NET INCOME $_____

(2) Subtract   FIXED MONTHLY EXPENSES: $_____

(3) Subtract   PERIODIC EXPENSES: $_____

(4) Subtract   DISCRETIONARY EXPENSES: $_____

YOUR *FINANCIAL FITNESS* IS

TOTAL $ ☺ (+) = **Happiness**

TOTAL $ ☹ (-) = **Sadness**

While this is only a sketchy, simplified version of the state of your monthly FINANCIAL FITNESS, - it does give you some idea of where your money is going. Most accountants and financial planners would agree that, if monthly expenses exceed monthly income, you have to immediately examine your discretionary spending habits. To get back on track, they would probably tell you to significantly reduce, or put a hold on, discretionary spending. Money saved through reductions in this one area will go a long way towards balancing your budget.

Next, you have to take a realistic look at your periodic expenses. Are you spending too much on utilities? telephone bill? gourmet food? snacks? alcoholic beverages? or designer clothes? Do you really need two phones? Realistically, many of the expenses in this category can be reduced, if you only put your mind to it. The savings could be used to start a tax-deferred retirement account.

Let's take a few moments to examine some ways to reduce spending

Let's start at the Supermarket. Your wife gave you a list of things to buy. You're walking down the aisle as your appetite center screams out, *'Get me some Mallomars...I Really Need Some Mallomars.'* If you're one of those palate-pleasers that listens to what your taste buds tell you - into the cart go the Mallomars. Next stop some potato chips, dips and Doritos. Don't worry if they're not on the list, your wife won't mind. Even if she does, they're already home and she wouldn't send you back to the store, would she? Now, all that's left on my wife's list; some milk, string beans, tomatoes and toilet paper and we're off to the cash register.

Stop right there! Look in the shopping cart. How many of those items were not on the list. Most people would readily admit that they spend too much money on snacks and prepared foods. What they generally don't realize is that, not only are these foods unhealthy to eat, they're equally bad for your budget. By strictly limiting your unhealthy snack purchases, you will not only take an important step towards *Getting Back to BASICS* - you will also save a lot of money.

I can't believe it. After all you've heard about the dangers of smoking, I can see you stopping by the cigarette vending machine. How can you do this to yourself? What did your lungs ever do to you? Except, work hard to keep you alive. All I can say is, *'if the human body was designed with a window in its chest, so that people would be able to look in a mirror and see their lung tissue, I suspect there would be far fewer smokers.'* Unfortunately, while everyone knows the dangers of smoking, so many of us don't heed the warning and will pay the price. The price is over $7.00 a pack now, and the prospect of lung cancer in the future - a double whammy.

Did you know that if you smoked just one pack of cigarettes a day you would have to shell out over TWENTY-FIVE HUNDRED DOLLARS each year just to cater to this unhealthy habit? When you make the big time and you're smoking two packs a day, you'll be wasting over FIVE THOUSAND DOLLARS of NET INCOME (*that's after taxes*) from your budget each year. By giving up this unhealthy habit, you'll greatly improve your health and go along way towards balancing your budget.

To Stay Healthy

Manage Your Money Wisely

And Don't Smoke!

> You're on the way home, driving your hi-octane gas-guzzler, when suddenly out of the corner of your eye; you spot a really nice pair of shoes in the window of your favorite designer clothes shop. You decide to stop, just for a moment, to see how much they cost.

When you find out, you almost pass out, but something in the back of your mind says, you must have them. You reach into your pocket to get some cash and your hand comes out holding lint. At that moment, you realize that you spent almost all of your available cash at the Supermarket. Before you get a chance to turn and leave, you try one last pocket and you find that all-important plastic card. You know, the one that says, *'you can have it now - even if you can't afford it.'* As you slap the card down on the counter, you don't give your budget a fleeting thought. As you leave the store, you feel good that you bought those expensive shoes, not realizing that on the upcoming bill-paying day, you'll pay in more ways than one, for this act of impulse buying.

Most of us have been guilty of impulse buying at one time or another. However, in order to get a handle on your finances, you must control your urge to spend. Remember, I spoke about how most people could not avoid eating blueberry pie if it's in the house. I told you that the key word was availability. I said if it's available you'll eat it. Well, the same philosophy applies to impulse buying. If you walk around with a lot of cash or credit cards in your pocket, you'll use them, whether you truly need the merchandise or not. To limit impulse buying it's a good idea to carry only $15.00 or $20.00 in your wallet above what you intend to spend on necessities. If you're off to the grocery store for milk and eggs, don't carry $200.00 cash and 6 credit cards in your wallet. That's a recipe for disaster.

In today's economy, perhaps more than ever – we must carefully review our spending habits.

The Impact Of Today's Economy On Your Health

If you think the 2009 economic crisis is hurting only your pocketbook, think again. Researchers say the decline of Wall Street, the mortgage crisis, and the looming threat of layoffs may take a heavy toll on your heart especially if you are already at risk for cardiac problems.

According to Louise Hawkley, PhD, associate director of the Social Neuroscience Laboratory at the University of Chicago, *'Financial stress can cause your whole cardiovascular system to be off. Elevated stress hormones constrict the blood vessels and create a vicious cycle where blood scrapes the cells and aggravates atherosclerotic plaque, which increases your risk for a cardiovascular event.'*

According to Redford Williams, MD, professor of psychiatry and behavioral sciences at Duke University, *'financial stress contributes to behavior proven to increase heart disease risk.'*

- Smokers are 13% less likely to quit during economic hard times.
- Ex-smokers are more likely to relapse.
- Drinkers tend to drink more, which drives up blood pressure.
- Alcoholics who have quit drinking are more prone to relapse.
- People eat less heart-healthy foods during times of stress

'So what do you do if the bad economy has you worried about your ticker? Dr. Williams cautions, first off, *'try not to panic. Take stock of your own situation and make sure you are not panicked about something that hasn't happened yet. But if your situation is dire, it's crucial not to isolate yourself. Sharing concerns with friends and getting social support can make your stress hormones go down and improve your health.'*

It's too early to judge the full impact on personal health caused by the current recession. However, it appears that because of the current economic meltdown many more Americans will suffer from stress-related illness and chronic disease.

To Survive The Economic Crisis With Your Health Intact

- Focus on *Getting Back to <u>Basics</u>*
- Maintain a good support system (*i.e. family, friends*)
- Take stock of your situation honestly
- Set solution-oriented realistic goals
- Make no excuses and work towards your stated goals
- Find ways to De-Stress

By now you know there is a strong relationship between money problems and health problems. The purpose of this chapter was not to teach you how to manage your money, but rather to present the idea that money problems are often the root cause of health problems. By learning how to live within your means during this very stressful time, you go a long way towards improving your health and taking another necessary step towards …

Getting Back to *<u>BASICS</u>*.

'Success is the sum of small efforts …
Repeated day in and day out.'
Robert Collier

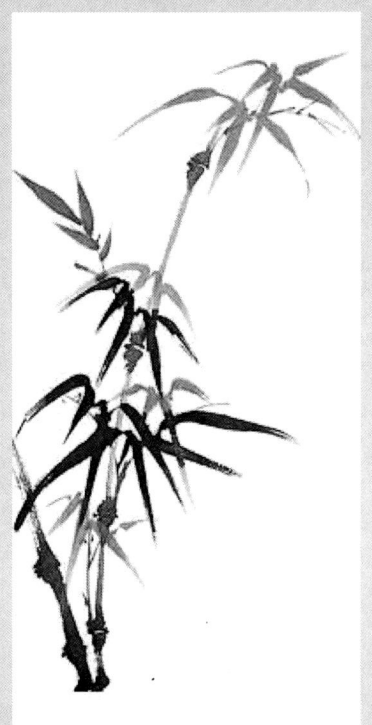

Part 8

Putting The Pieces Together

There Are No Excuses

So Now You Know

A Moment of Clarity

Sometimes in life, we have *moments of clarity* where everything seems to make sense. At those brief, fleeting times, we may come to realize that the responsibility for the way we live is ultimately in our own hands. What was yesterday does not have to be our tomorrow. Our destiny can be a new beginning that leads to a brighter future. As we move from what was familiar yesterday into unfamiliar territory, we must accept that - as our world is changing – so must we. As we adjust to the new reality, we take the final positive step towards …

Getting Back to <u>BASICS</u>.

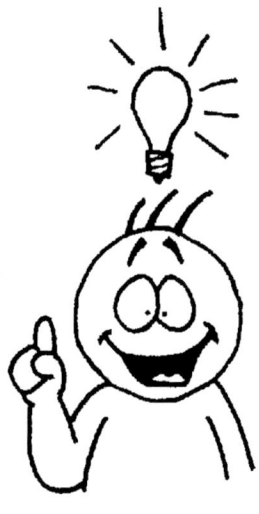

I Got It

There Are No Excuses

> 'I believe anyone can conquer fear
> by doing the things they fear to do,
> provided they keep doing them
> until they get a record of successful
> experiences behind them.'
>
> -*Eleanor Roosevelt*-

We all have fears. They may be things that we find unpleasant to do, situations we try our best to avoid and things, like spiders or snakes, that may frighten us. However, these words of Eleanor Roosevelt I interpret to mean you can't be afraid to try new things. You can't live life paralyzed by the fear of change. <u>Success only comes to those who conquer their fears by facing up to them.</u>

For whatever reason, you've taken some of your valuable time to read this book. Up to this point you may have found some portions humorous, some informative, and you might even have found some parts entertaining. I wouldn't be surprised if you agree with some of the things I've said. However, agreeing with me and putting some of the ideas I present into action are two completely different matters.

This brings up an interesting story. A friend of mine recently complained that he was having difficulty getting to sleep and staying asleep. I thought for a moment and said to myself, here's a perfect test to determine if some of the things I write about truly benefit others. I told him that it might be a good idea for him to read my book and pay particularly close attention to the chapter on how to sleep soundly. One week later, he stopped by at the office to thank me for my help. Of course, being one week later, I had completely forgotten our previous conversation and asked him what he was thanking me for. In hindsight, I should have said, '*you're welcome,*' but I didn't and soon paid the price. He went on to explain that he took my advice about getting to sleep and found that it worked.'

'*What advice worked?*' I inquired.
'*You know, to read your book.*'
'*How did it help?*' I asked.
And he replied,

'*As soon as I started reading your book -* <u>*I fell asleep.*</u>'

As you can see, I've found that in order to stay balanced in life, you can't take yourself too seriously. You have to be able to poke fun at yourself, and whenever possible, look for the humorous side of life.

In case you're taking yourself too seriously right about now, I thought it would be a good idea to relate another bit of humor I recently found on the Internet. It was listed under the heading:

To Exercise Or Not To Exercise
Author Unknown

- It is well documented that for every mile you jog, you add one minute to your life. This enables you, at age 85, to spend an additional 5 months in a nursing home at $5,000 per month.

- My grandmother started walking 5 miles a day when she was 60. Now she's 97 and we don't know where the heck she is.

- The only reason I would take up jogging is so that I could hear heavy breathing again,

- I joined a health club last year, spent about $400. Haven't lost a pound. Apparently you have to show up.

- I have to exercise early in the morning before my brain has figured out what I'm doing.

- I don't exercise at all. If G-d meant us to touch our toes, he would have put them further up our body.

- I like long walks, especially when taken by people who annoy me.

- I have flabby thighs, but fortunately my stomach covers them.

- I don't jog - it makes the ice jump right out of my glass.

- And finally - If you are going to try cross-country skiing, start with a small country.

You have to admit, that's pretty funny stuff. Regrettably, many of those exercise excuses are not so far fetched. In fact, over the years I've heard some pretty inventive excuses. Listed below are some of the more creative ones.

Excuses Not To Exercise

- I never have the time to exercise
- I'm too tired to exercise
- I'm too old to exercise
- I get enough exercise at work - I'm a dental hygienist
- I don't care how I look - so why exercise
- It's boring
- My car broke down so I couldn't get to the gym
- The toilets at the gym are disgusting
- I'm perfect just the way I am
- It's too hard
- It's too easy
- I know it's good for me - but I just don't like it
- My astrologist said it's not a good day to workout
- I just got my nails done - so I can't exercise this week
- The dog ate my sneakers
- I have a headache
- It's too expensive to join a gym
- I don't look good in gym clothes
- Wearing sneakers ruins a good pedicure
- I hate to sweat
- I like to sweat - but not by exercising
- It's against my religion
- I take a pill - anytime I get the urge to exercise
- My treadmill is really a clotheshorse in disguise
- My gym doesn't allow cellular phones
- I tried it once
- Hey, I'm already married - so why do I have to look good
- I'd rather be fishing
- I'd rather be _____ (fill in the blank)

I guess it's all in the way you look at things. If you're a pessimist, the glass is always half empty. If you're an optimist, the glass is always half filled. Instead of looking for excuses not to exercise, let's turn that idea around and examine some good reasons to exercise.

Good Reasons To Exercise

- It makes me feel better
- It makes me healthier
- It's a great social activity
- I meet new people
- My body feels great after a workout
- It helps me lose weight
- It helps me control my weight
- I'm no longer depressed
- It's nice to keep up with the grandchildren
- I look and feel younger
- I have more strength and stamina
- I handle stress a lot better
- My energy level is way up there
- It helps me remain independent
- I get some time to think
- I like to sweat
- I eat less and I eat healthier
- I feel powerful
- I feel refreshed
- I feel energetic and empowered
- My dog loves to go for long walks
- I don't feel like a sedentary, pencil pusher
- Those endorphins make me feel great

Are you one of those people who make New Years resolutions to lose weight or begin exercising that are broken by April 1st? Well, in case you didn't know it, you're not alone. Approximately 50% of all serious New Years resolutions are broken within the first three months.

Let's take a moment to discuss why one person quits a lifestyle improvement program, and another keeps going. I frequently have clients tell me how they started and stopped going to this program or that. Program compliance is traditionally quite low in health club, weight loss and wellness programs. Even the noted author, Mark Twain, poked fun at our propensity to not follow-through when he said,

'I can stop smoking anytime I want – I've done it a thousand times.'

So what could I possibly say to make you really want to change your life, maintain a healthier lifestyle - and keep it up?

Do It Because You Need To!

I can't say it any louder than that - at least not on this page. Those six words should be motivation enough to get you started. You know that you have to change. Your doctor, family and friends are counting on you to get healthy - and stay healthy. Now it's up to you.

Hopefully by now you've made the decision to begin making some sensible and healthful changes. All I have to do now is convince you to keep it up. Based on current statistics, which say 50% of you will quit by April 1st, that's no easy task. However, I've never been one to shy away from a challenge, and neither should you. My challenge is to say something, which will motivate you to make changes in your life. Yours is to build the strength, determination, will power, perseverance, and commitment - (*call it whatever you'd like*) - to make it happen.

Before you begin your quest to get healthy - and stay healthy, I'd like to talk about a word that most of us have come to dread since our earliest days in grammar school. That word is - *failure*. As soon as I think of the word *failure*, I think of the words:

d--e--f--e--a--t

m--i--s--t--a--k--e

s--h--a--m--e

d--i--s--a--p--p--o--i--n--t--m--e--n--t

f--r--u--s--t--r--a--t--i--o--n

f--l--a--w

i--n--a--d--e--q--u--a--c--y

What you have to remember before you go any further is that when you make the decision to change, you have to put everything into that decision. The word failure should not exist in your vocabulary. I repeat the word failure should not exist. If you begin any program, or creative endeavor, with the word failure lurking out there in the wings - it will sap your strength, weaken your resolve - and diminish your passion for success. Eleanor Roosevelt was right when she said, 'I believe anyone can conquer fear by doing the things they fear to do.' If you focus on success and don't consider failure an option - you will succeed.

Another equally important thing to remember is - you have to believe that you can succeed. Don't limit your self-image by saying, *I'm fat - and I'm always going to be fat,* or *'I tried to stop smoking, but I don't have the will power.'* You have to believe in yourself. There are no limitations to what you can do if you truly want to do it. The only limitations are those our minds create when we have fear of failure.

And finally, in order for you to strive for success and believe in yourself you have to create a lot of positive self-talk. We have to convince ourselves, sort of from the inside out; that what we're doing is good for us, healthy for us. Phrases like *I can* and *I will* help to build self-esteem and internally motivate you towards success.

Whenever you feel the urge to quit, remember

'I believe anyone can conquer fear
by doing the things they fear to do,
provided they keep doing them
until they get a record of successful
experiences behind them.'

-Eleanor Roosevelt-

So now it's up to you!

You can choose to do nothing

and just let things happen …

or

You can choose to

take control of your life,

and

Get Back to BASICS.

So Now You Know

As I bring this book to a close, I expect that some of you may disagree with some of my ideas. I neither seek nor expect unanimous approval. However, <u>I believe that many of you will benefit greatly if you begin to make positive lifestyle changes</u>. Whether or not those ideas came from this book or some other source is irrelevant. What is relevant is that, you have taken some action to improve your life and health.

So now you know that there are things you can do to improve your health and make your life more enjoyable. However, there is one word of caution. Believe it or not, the word is <u>social</u>.

By nature, humans are social animals. We have a need to interact with others. It is this need that occasionally causes us to do things, which might not be good for us. Often, societal pressures influence our decisions. While we might not ordinarily smoke, drink or overeat, in a group setting this may not be the case. Often times, well-intentioned friends or relatives may ask you to join them for a drink, have a smoke or eat a donut. Sometimes the offer is made because they need your approval to validate their own unhealthy habits. Our culture is so wrapped up in social etiquette, that to refuse their offer may be deemed an insult.

What you have to remember is <u>when you first begin a program of lifestyle improvement, it's almost as if you're sitting on a fence</u>. Fall one-way and you get healthy. Fall the other way and you don't. The first four to six weeks are the most difficult. Your body is changing, improvements are being made, but you can't see them. As I told you before, all the good stuff is taking place at the cellular level and would require an electron microscope to observe. It's during this fragile four to six week period that most people give up.

Time and time again, patients and friends have shared their concern about social functions where they tend to over-indulge. Often they tell me that they have no willpower to control themselves. As soon as I hear this, I think of the 16-year old who may be pressured to illegally smoke or drink by their peers. At that age the pressure is pretty intense. All I can say is, *'we're not sixteen anymore. You don't have to give in to social pressures to do things that you know are not good for you. <u>You've reached a stage in life where you can just say no!</u> - <u>in a polite way</u>.'*

Over the years, I've always been intrigued by the fact that, while most of us know that we have to eat right, exercise and make positive lifestyle choices in order to stay healthy, so many of us end up in poor shape as we get older. Perhaps the reason for this has something to do with the <u>Concept of Responsibility</u>.

You know - <u>Responsibility for</u> ...

- Developing a career

- Managing a household

- Raising children

- Paying bills

- Providing food and shelter for our family

- Dealing with aged parents

As we get older, get married, have children and take on more responsibilities in our lives, we make sacrifices. While these sacrifices may be helpful for our families, they may not always be good for our health. Most of us would agree that it's not uncommon for parents to overwork or deny themselves for the sake of their children. However, parents must understand that <u>parenting is a lifelong responsibility</u>. By denying themselves the <u>Basics</u> for maintaining good health, they may ultimately shorten their lives.

It's interesting to note that many of you have spent your entire adult life in the pursuit of money, so that you will be able to provide for your family and enjoy your retirement years. Unfortunately, many successful people don't live long enough to retire. They worked hard to <u>Build Wealth</u> - <u>Not Health</u>. And while I have nothing against being successful, you must remember that <u>the number one priority in life must be good health.</u>

<u>Consider this interesting Paradox</u>

> We strive for <u>Wealth</u>
>
> At the expense of our <u>Health</u>,
>
> Then use our <u>Wealth</u>
>
> Attempting to regain our <u>Health</u>

If you think of life in these terms, it's almost like a dog chasing it's own tail. Right about now, I'm long overdue for a workout. This miracle baby knows that while some people with good genes may do everything wrong and still appear to be healthy and robust, most of us have to make a personal commitment to stay healthy.

We all have choices in life, decisions to make, which will affect the outcome of how we feel and possibly how long we live. The road you are about to begin will not always be easy to navigate. There will be many external pressures and *nay Sayers* along the way that, for whatever reason, may not want you to achieve your goal. Just remember, in spite of the obstacles if you stay motivated – you can succeed!

As our world is changing, so must we. Our challenge is to prepare ourselves mentally and physically to handle the stressors of the new reality. You've reached a crucial stage in your life at a critical time in our country. Right now you're sitting on a fence. Fall forward to the future and you become healthier. Fall backwards to the past and your unhealthy habits may soon catch up with you and bite you on your behind.

The time has come to live

healthier, *happier* and possibly *longer* by …

GETTING BACK TO BASICS

*'Make the decision to change today!
You learn from a decision ...
You learn nothing from indecision'*

Unknown

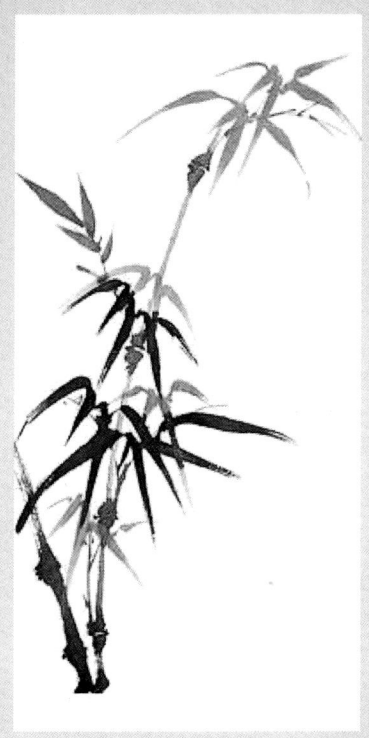

Appendix A

Resistance-Training Program

Resistance-Training Program

> The following pages contain illustrations and descriptions of dumbbell weight training exercises that I have found work well for most people just beginning to exercise. Before you begin, I suggest that you read the chapter: *Sensible Guidelines for Resistance Training* beginning on page 51.

Resistance-Training Guidelines

- Begin with a very low weight
- Do not exercise the same muscles every day
- Lift weights with slow, controlled movement
- When you lift a weight do not hold your breath
- Stay well hydrated
- Do not ignore symptoms of intolerance

CAUTION

If you're just beginning to exercise, or have any physical condition that might be affected by resistance training, speak with your doctor before you start.

Resistance Training
Exercise: *Bicep Curl*

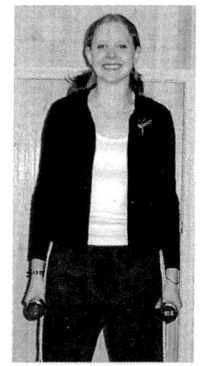

Position [1] • Starting position with palms facing hips.

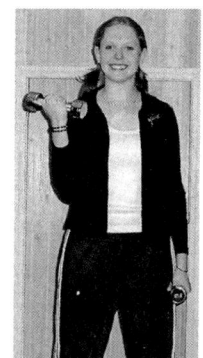

Position [2] • Lift right hand and rotate palm facing shoulder.

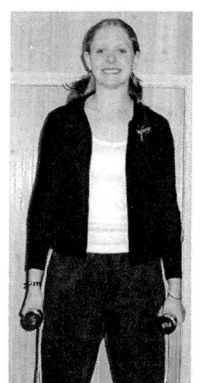

Position [3] • Return to starting position rotating palms facing hips.

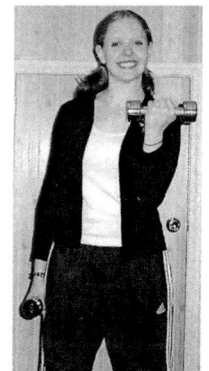

Position [4] • Lift left hand and rotate palm facing shoulder.

Starting Position: Weights held at side of body with palms facing hips. Feet comfortably separated with knees slightly bent.

Movement: Lift right hand to right shoulder while rotating palm to face your shoulder. Lower right hand to your side while rotating palm to face your hip. Repeat with your left hand to complete one repetition of this exercise.

Things to remember:
Count 1/1 – 2/2 – 3/3 etc. as you lift each arm to keep track of your reps.
Do not do more than 12 reps of this exercise the first time.
Use slow, controlled movements in both directions
Breathe out as you lift the weight. DO NOT HOLD YOUR BREATH.
If you're just beginning a weight-training program – start with a low weight.

Resistance Training
Exercise: *Seated Press*

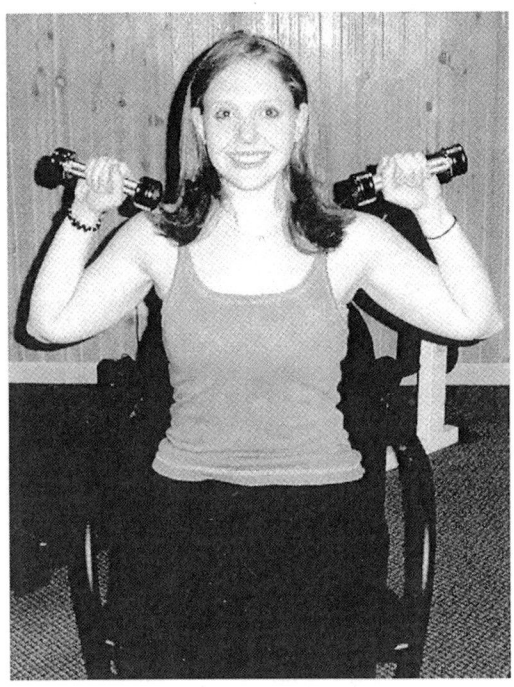

Position [1] • Starting position

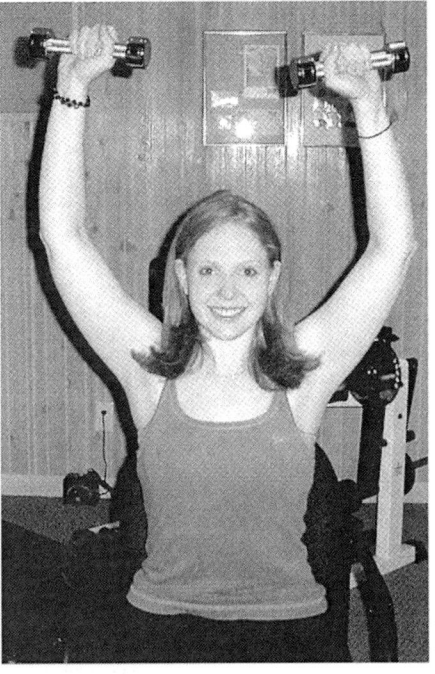

Position [2] • Lift weight slowly and breathe out. Do not lock out your elbows.

Starting Position: Seated in a straight back chair with good back support. Weights held by your shoulders with palms facing forward.

Movement: Lift both weights at the same time – but do not lock out your elbows. Lower the weights to complete one repetition of this exercise.

Things to remember:
Count 1-2-3 etc. as you lift both arms to keep track of your reps.
Do not do more than 12 reps of this exercise the first time.
Use slow, controlled movements in both directions
Breathe out as you lift the weight. DO NOT HOLD YOUR BREATH.
If you're just beginning a weight-training program – start with a low weight.

Resistance Training
Exercise: *French Curl*

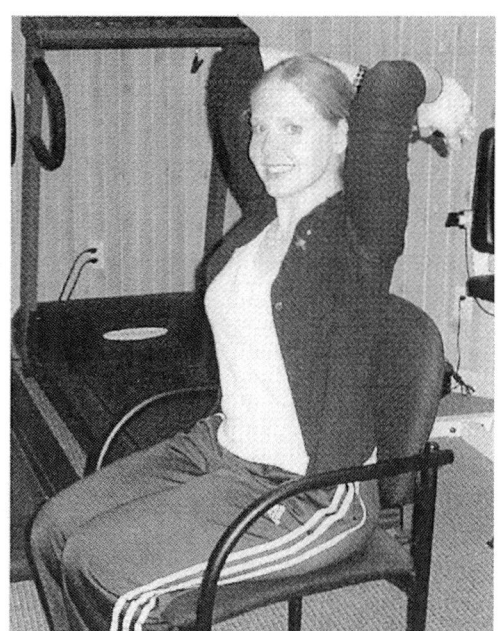

Position [1] • Starting position

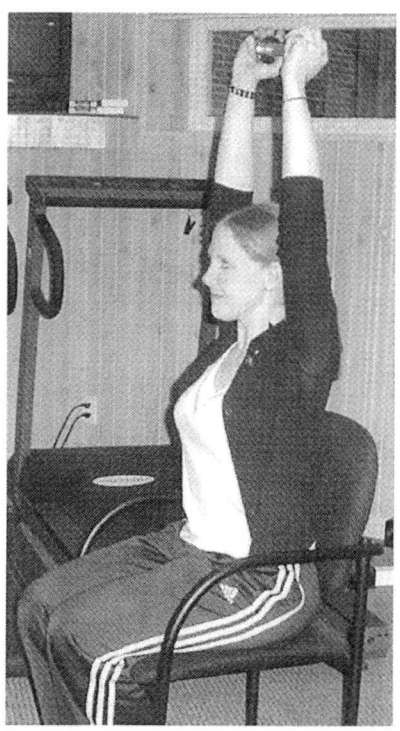

Position [2] • Lift weights slowly over your head and breathe out. Do not lock out your elbows.

Starting Position: Seated in a straight back chair with good back support. Use only one dumbbell weight for this exercise. Grip the weight at each end positioning the weight behind your head.

Movement: Lift the weight slowly towards the ceiling. Do not lock out your elbows. Lower the weight behind your head to complete one repetition of this exercise.

Things to remember:
Count 1-2-3 etc. as you lift the weight over head to keep track of your reps.
Do not do more than 12 reps of this exercise the first time.
Use slow, controlled movements in both directions
Breathe out as you lift the weight. DO NOT HOLD YOUR BREATH.
If you're just beginning a weight-training program – start with a low weight.

Resistance Training
Exercise: *High Pull*

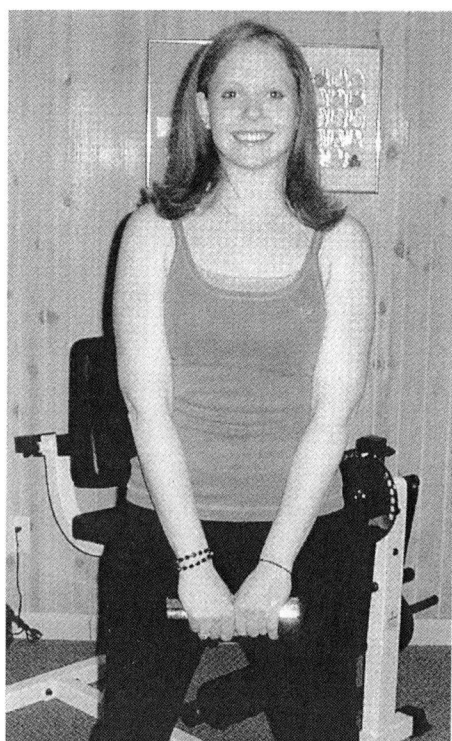
Position [1] • Starting position

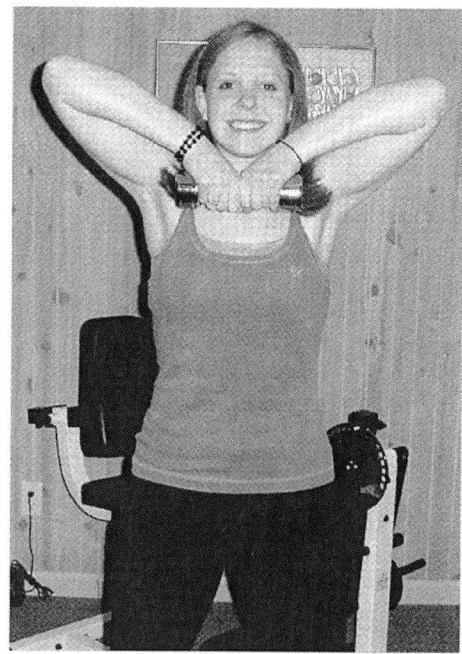
Position [2] • Lift weights under Chin with elbows flared out.

<u>Starting Position</u>: Use only one weight for this exercise. While standing, grip the weight in the middle (*Refer to illustration*) with both hands. Position the weight below your waist. Feet comfortably separated with knees slightly bent.

<u>Movement</u>: Lift the weight straight up under your chin as you flare your elbows to the side. Lower the weight to the staring position to complete one repetition of this exercise.

<u>Things to remember</u>:
Count 1-2-3 etc. as you lift the weight up to keep track of your reps.
Do not do more than 12 reps of this exercise the first time.
Use slow, controlled movements in both directions
Breathe out as you lift the weight. DO NOT HOLD YOUR BREATH.
If you're just beginning a weight-training program – start with a low weight.

Resistance Training
Exercise: *Bent Row*

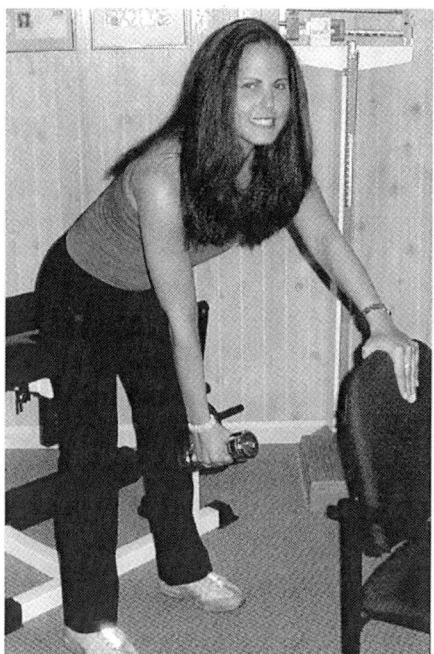

Position [1] • Starting position

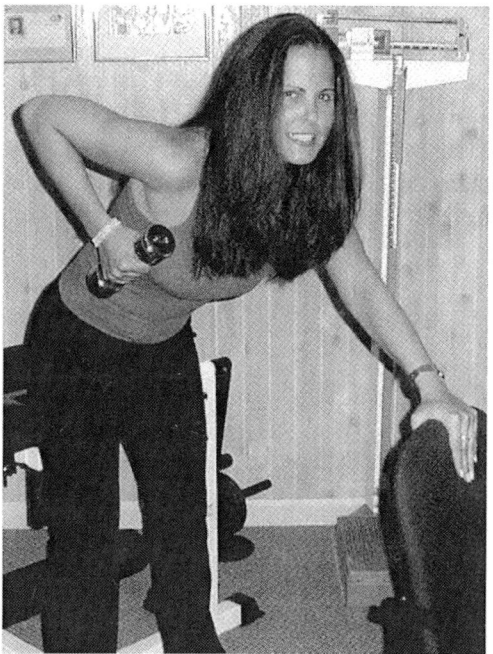

Position [2] • Lift weight close to armpit then return to starting position.

Starting Position: Stand behind a stable chair. Position your feet in line with the chair legs approximately two feet behind the chair. Bend forward and place your left hand in the middle of the back support, keeping your weight evenly balanced. Position the weight in your right hand directly below your body. (*Refer to illustration*)

Movement: Lift the weight in your right hand towards your armpit, flaring your elbow outwards. Lower the weight to the starting position to complete one rep. After you complete 12 reps with your right hand – change hand position (right hand holding the chair) and repeat the same exercise with your left hand.

Things to remember:
Count 1-2-3 etc. as you lift the weight to keep track of your reps.
Do not do more than 12 reps of this exercise the first time.
Use slow, controlled movements in both directions
Breathe out as you lift the weight. DO NOT HOLD YOUR BREATH.
If you're just beginning a weight-training program – start with a low weight.

Resistance Training
Exercise: *Tricep Extension*

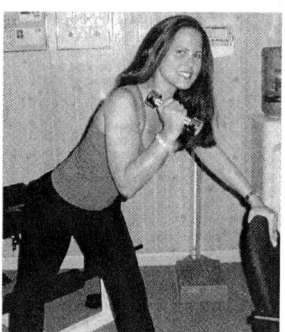

Position [1] • Starting position

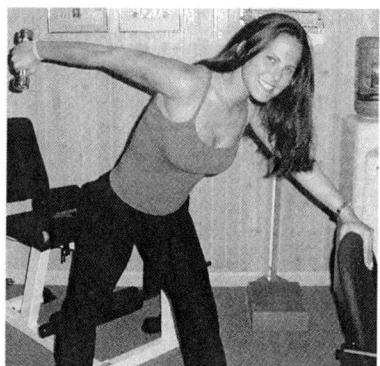

Position [2] • Arc weight backwards then arc forward to starting position

Starting Position: Place your left foot 12-18 inches behind a stable chair. Position your right foot two feet behind your left foot. Bend forward and place your left hand on the middle of the back support distributing your weight evenly. Hold the weight in your right hand by your shoulder. (*Refer to illustration*)

Movement: Slowly arc the weight backwards being careful not to over-extend. Arc the weight forward to the starting position to complete one repetition of this exercise.

Things to remember:
Count 1-2-3 etc. as you arc the weight backwards to keep track of your reps.
Do not do more than 12 reps of this exercise the first time.
Use slow, controlled movements in both directions
Breathe out as you lift the weight. DO NOT HOLD YOUR BREATH.
If you're just beginning a weight-training program – start with a low weight.

Resistance Training
Exercise: *Chest Press*

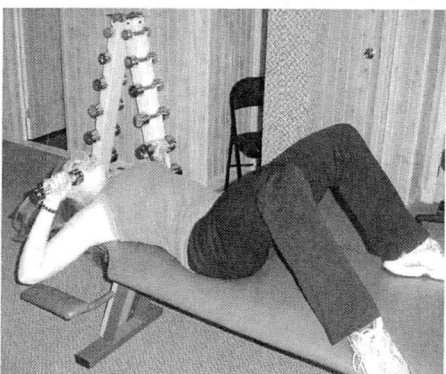

Position [1] • Starting position

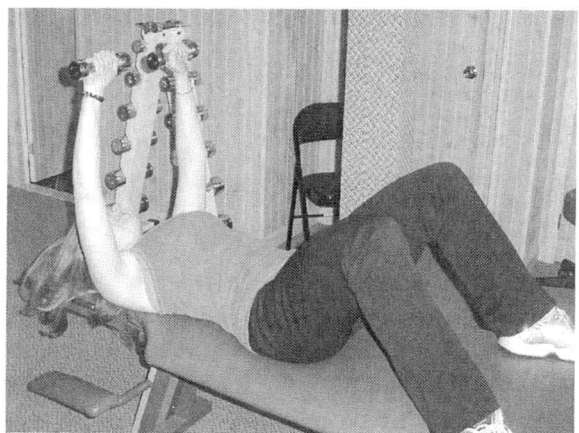

Position [2] • Lift weights but do not lock out elbows - then return to starting position.

Starting Position: Lying on your back on a flat bench with knees flexed. Hold dumbbell weights in line with your chest at a right angle. *(Refer to illustration)*

Movement: Lift the weight slowly towards the ceiling. Do not lock out your elbows. Lower the weight to the starting position to complete one repetition of this exercise.

Things to remember:
Count 1-2-3 etc. as you lift the weights up to keep track of your reps.
Do not do more than 12 reps of this exercise the first time.
Use slow, controlled movements in both directions
Breathe out as you lift the weight. DO NOT HOLD YOUR BREATH.
If you're just beginning a weight-training program – start with a low weight.

Resistance Training
Exercise: *Lying Pullover*

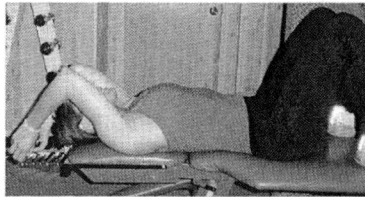
Position [1] • Weight behind and below head

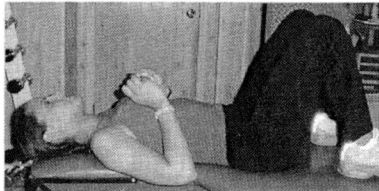
Position [4] • Move weight towards head

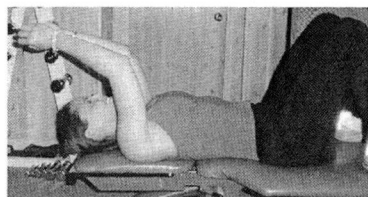
Position [2] • Arc weight forward

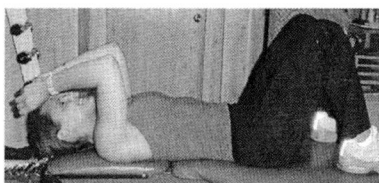
Position [5] • Weight moves over head

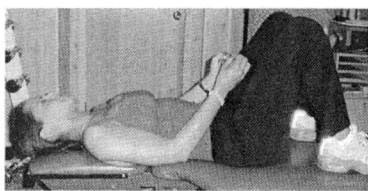
Position [3] • Arc weight to pelvis

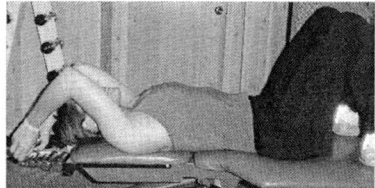
Position [6] • Return to starting position

Starting Position: Use one weight for this exercise. Lying on your back on a flat bench with knees flexed. Hold the weight at both ends *(Refer to illustration)* positioned behind and below your head.

Movement: Arc the weight slowly over your head to above your pelvis. Draw the weight forward across your body towards your head. Lower the weight behind and below your head to complete one repetition of this exercise

Things to remember:
Count 1-2-3 etc. as you arc the weight forward to keep track of your reps.
Do not do more than 12 reps of this exercise the first time.
Use slow, controlled movements in both directions
Breathe out as you lift the weight. DO NOT HOLD YOUR BREATH.
If you're just beginning a weight-training program – start with a low weight.

Resistance Training
Exercise: *Abdominal Curl*

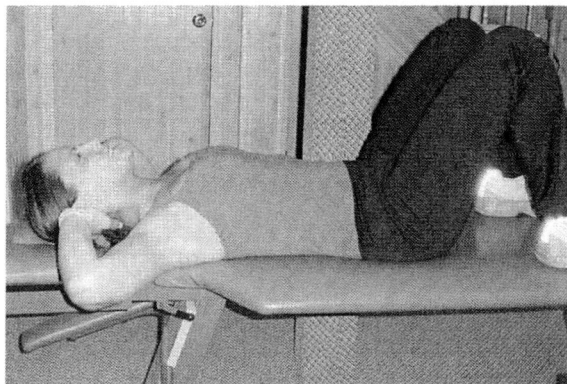

Position [1] • Starting position

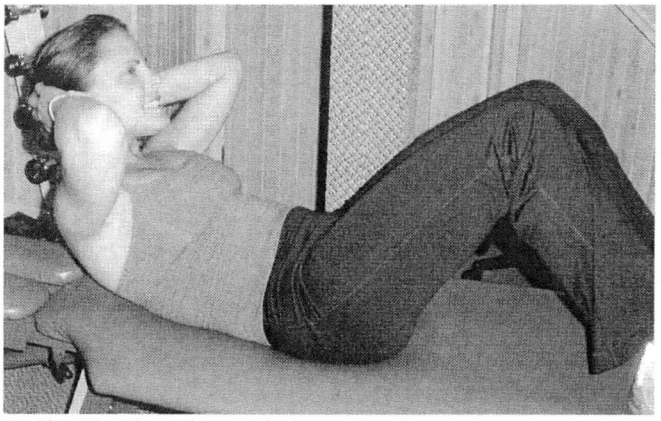

Position [2] • Lift shoulders 2-4 inches and breathe out - then return to starting position. Make sure to keep knees bent.

Starting Position: Lying on your back on a flat bench or carpeted surface with knees flexed. Hands may be clasped behind your neck or folded across your chest.

Movement: Take a breath before you start. Tuck your chin to your chest and round your shoulders as you gently lift your shoulders 2-4 inches off the surface as your breathe out. Gently lower your body to complete one repetition of this exercise.

Things to remember:
Count 1-2-3 as you lift your body to keep track of your reps.
Do not do more than 12-15 reps of this exercise the first time.
Use slow, controlled movements in both directions.

Resistance Training
Exercise: *Inner Thigh - Adduction*

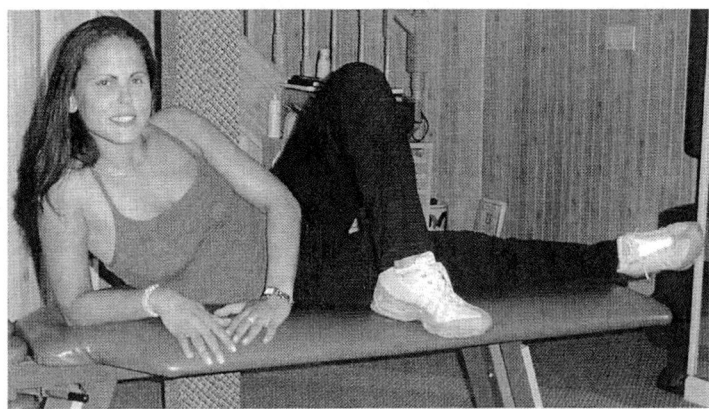
Position [1] • Starting position

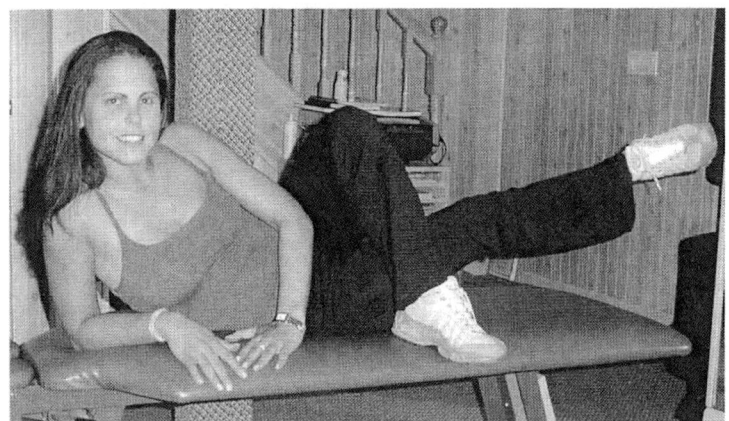
Position [2] • Lift lower leg slowly then return to starting position.

Starting Position: Lying on your side on a flat bench or carpeted surface. Extend your lower leg straight out. Position your upper leg in front of your body as shown in the illustration.

Movement: Gently lift your lower leg to a comfortable height. Do not throw your leg up. Slowly lower your leg to the starting position to complete one repetition of this exercise.

Things to remember:
Count 1-2-3 as you lift your leg to keep track of your reps.
Do not do more than 12-15 reps of this exercise the first time.
Use slow, controlled movements in both directions.

Resistance Training
Exercise: *Outer Thigh - Abduction*

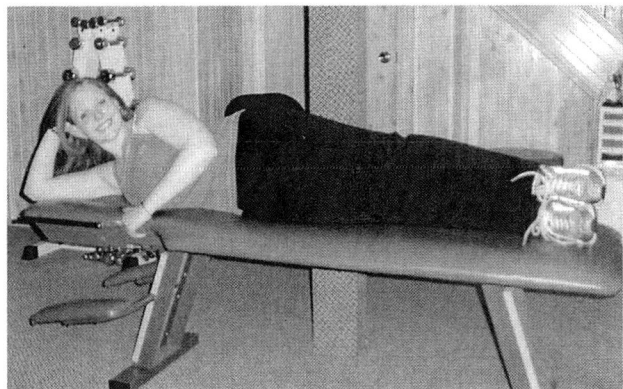
Position [1] • Starting position

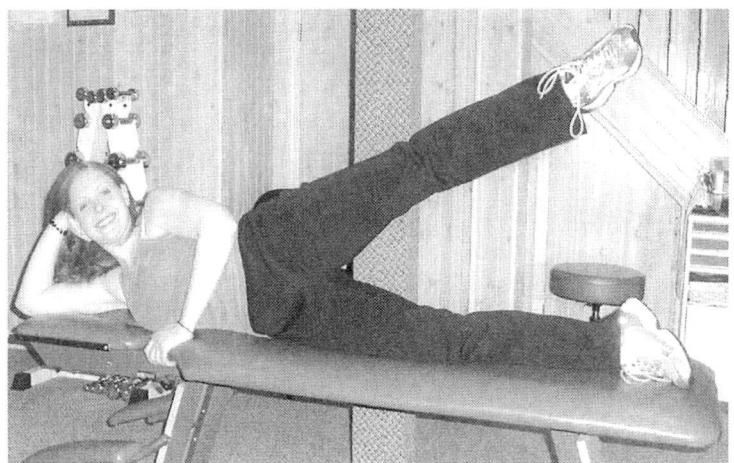
Position [2] • Lift upper leg slowly then return to starting position.

Starting Position: Lying on your side on a flat bench or carpeted surface. Extend both legs straight out with one leg on top of the other *(Refer to illustration)*

Movement: Gently lift your upper leg to a comfortable height. Do not throw your leg up. Slowly lower your leg to the starting position to complete one repetition of this exercise.

Things to remember:
Count 1-2-3 as you lift your leg to keep track of your reps.
Do not do more than 12-15 reps of this exercise the first time.
Use slow, controlled movements in both directions

Resistance Training
Exercise: *Seated Leg Extension*

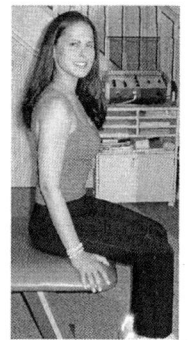
Position [1] • Starting position

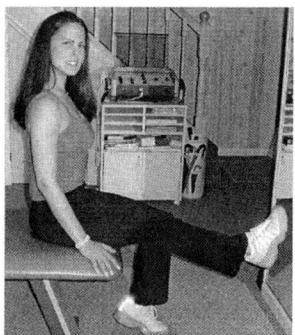
Position [2] • Lift right leg forwards then lower to starting position. Do each foot 5, 10 or 15 times

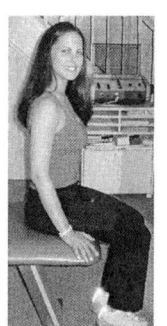
Position [1] • Starting position

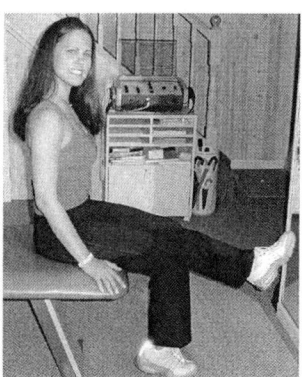
Position [2] • Do the same exercise for the left foot 5, 10 or 15 times. Do not throw the leg forward.

Starting Position: Seated comfortably in a stable chair with a straight back. *(Refer to illustration)*

Movement: gently lift your right leg to a comfortable height. Do not throw your leg up or hyper-extend to a locked out position. Gently lower your leg to the starting position to complete one repetition of this exercise. When you complete 12-15 reps with your right leg – repeat the same exercise with your left leg.

Things to remember:
Count 1-2-3 as you lift your leg to keep track of your reps.
Do not do more than 12-15 reps of this exercise the first time.
Use slow, controlled movements in both directions.
You can increase the difficulty of this exercise using light ankle weights.

Resistance Training
Exercise: *Standing Leg Curl*

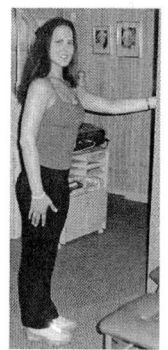

Position [1] • Starting position

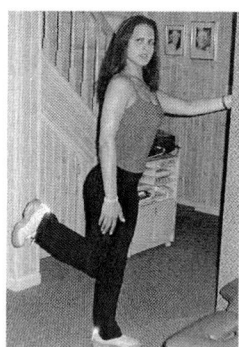

Position [2] • Lift right leg backwards then lower to starting position. Do each foot 5, 10 or 15 times.

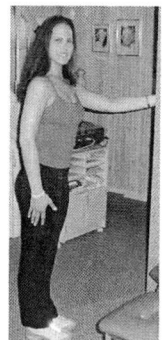

Position [1] • Starting position

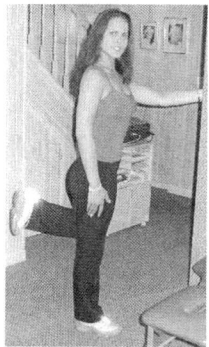

Position [2] • Do the same exercise for the left foot 5, 10 or 15 times. Do not throw the leg backwards.

Starting Position: Standing behind a stable chair with a straight back. Make sure to keep your back straight as you perform this exercise. *(Refer to illustration)*

Movement: Gently lift your right leg backwards to a comfortable height. Do not throw your leg backwards. Gently lower your leg to the starting position to complete one repetition of this exercise. When you complete 12-15 reps with your right leg – repeat the same exercise with your left leg.

Things to remember:
Count 1-2-3 as you lift your leg to keep track of your reps.
Do not do more than 12-15 reps of this exercise the first time.
Use slow, controlled movements in both directions.
You can increase the difficulty of this exercise using light ankle weights.

Quad Stretch

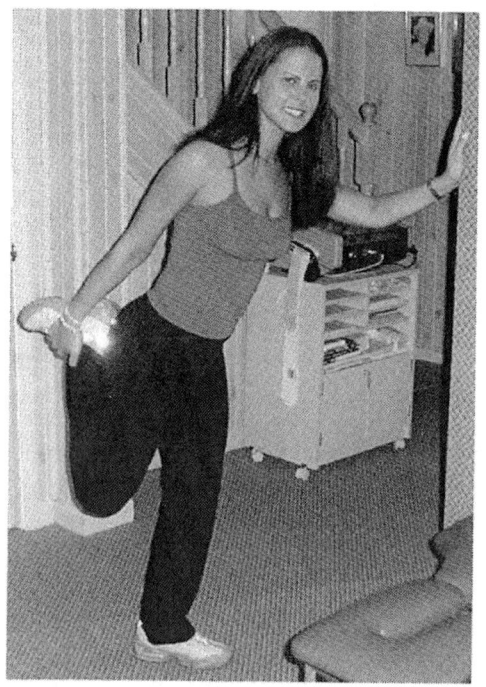

Right quad stretch

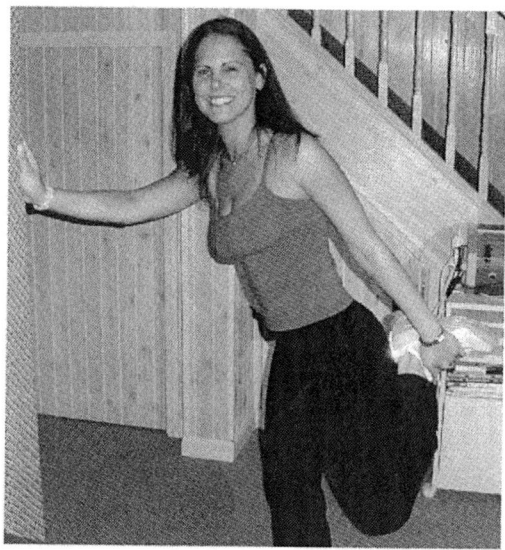

Left quad stretch

Starting Position: Standing holding onto a countertop (*or wall*) with your left hand. Carefully extend your right leg backwards and grab your right ankle with your right hand (*Refer to illustration*). If you have difficulty doing this, you may perform this exercise while lying on your side - on a carpeted surface.

Movement: Gently pull your right ankle up as your stretch to the point of slight discomfort (*Initial stage*). Hold the stretch for several seconds. If the discomfort '*melts away*' you may increase the stretch slightly (*Developmental stage*). Change position and repeat the stretch with your left leg.

Things to remember:
Do not bounce as you stretch.

Hamstring Stretch

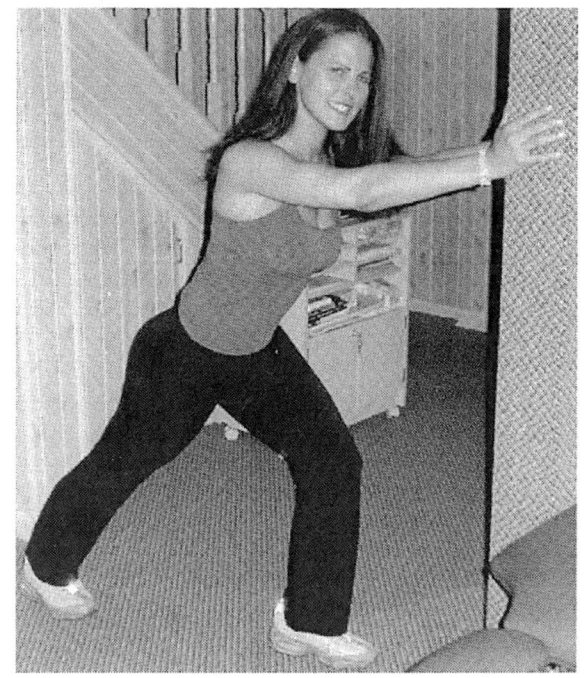

Right hamstring stretch

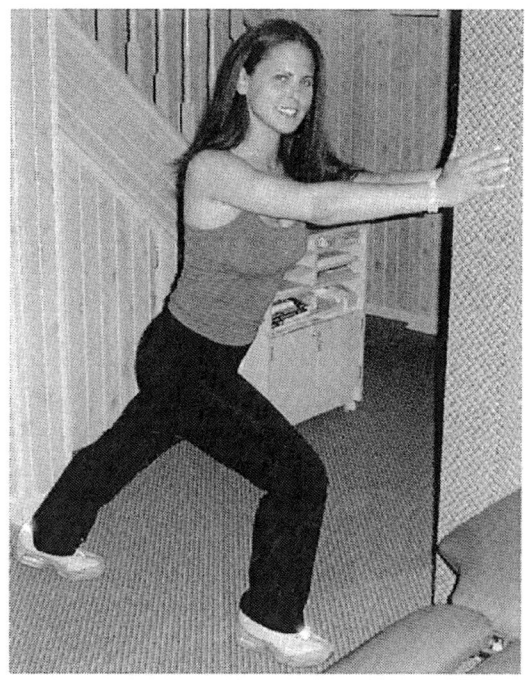

Left hamstring stretch

<u>Starting Position</u>: Stand and hold onto a countertop (*or wall*) with your left leg forward and your right leg behind. *(Refer to illustration)*

<u>Movement</u>: Gently press forward towards the wall as you feel the stretch on the back of your right thigh. Stretch to the point of slight discomfort (*Initial stage*). Hold the stretch for several seconds. If the discomfort '*melts away*' you may increase the stretch slightly (*Developmental stage*). Change position and repeat the stretch with your left leg.

To stretch your calf muscles - keep the heel of your rear foot planted firmly and slowly bend your rear leg. You should feel the stretch in your calf muscle below the knee. Stretch to the point of slight discomfort (*Initial stage*). Hold the stretch for several seconds. If the discomfort '*melts away*' you may increase the stretch slightly (*Developmental stage*). Change position and repeat the stretch with your other leg.

<u>Things to remember</u>:
Do not bounce as you stretch.

About the Author

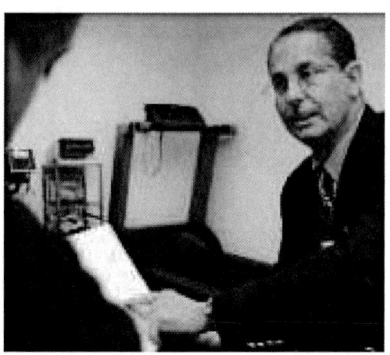

Barry M. Stein is a *Clinical Exercise Physiologist* with more than thirty years experience in corporate, commercial and medical fitness settings. He has authored four lifestyle improvement books and is currently assisting the North Shore LIJ Health System with the design of music videos as part of their pediatric obesity initiative. As President of *Get Fit For Life, LLC.* he developed the *True Age Test* available at *www.MyTrueAge.com*.

Additional Accomplishments:

President, Get Fit For Life, LLC. (1995-Present)

Faculty, Center for Weight Management, Department of Medicine, NSLIJ Health System (2003-2009)

Member, Wellness Advisory Committee, North Shore-LIJ Health System (2007-2009)

Clinical Exercise Physiologist, Department of Medicine – Long Island Jewish Medical Center (2003-2009)

Consultant/Designer, North Shore-LIJ Health System – '*Activity Works*' music videos (2008-2009)

Director, Laboratory of Applied Physiology, Cardiac Rehabilitation Center, Miami, Florida.

Research Physiologist, Health Risk Assessment Corporation, Los Angeles, CA.

New Product Development/Marketing Specialist, Upjohn HealthCare Services: A Division of The Upjohn Company, Kalamazoo, MI.

Curriculum Writer, (CUNY) City University of New York - Assisted in the design of the Exercise Science/Personal Training certificate and associate's degree program.

President, Lenbar Sports Medical, Designed PROFILE 1000 Wellness System and FAST TRACK Optical Scanning System. Negotiated product endorsement for PROFILE 1000 from Upjohn Healthcare Services.

National Program Director, (AACLSA) American Association of Clinical Laboratory Supervisors and Administrators. Developed programming in conjunction with the NYC Department of Health.

Vice President/ New Product Development/Marketing, Data Pep Associates, Inc. Fort Lee, New Jersey. Designed Sports Medicine computer applications for the Wang 2200 computer.

Founding Member, Bergen County Health and Fitness Council.

Applied Physiologist, American Sports Medical Training Center - Exercise Assessments and prescriptive exercise programming for Olympic athletes - USOC Sports Medicine Division.